T4-AKC-179

TO HAVE... TO HOLD...

A Parents' Guide to Childbirth & Early Parenting

Second Edition

by Joyce L. Kieffer, R.N., B.S., CCE

Training Resource Associates
Harrisburg, Pennsylvania

10 9 8 7 6 5 4 3 2 1

LIBRARY OF CONGRESS CATALOG CARD NO.: 80-54451

ISBN 0-933794-02-9

© TRAINING RESOURCE ASSOCIATES, MCMLXXXI All rights reserved.
This publication, or any parts thereof, may not be reproduced or transmitted in
any form or by any means, electronic or mechanical, including photocopying,
recording, storage in an information retrieval system, or otherwise, without the
express written permission of the publisher.

Design & Illustration by
Colonial Quill Associates, Gettysburg, Pa.

This manual is dedicated to all the unborn children whose birth and early years are made richer and more joyful because their parents read this book.

In *"TO HAVE . . . TO HOLD. . . ,"* Joyce L. Kieffer shares the knowledge and experience of her seventeen years in nursing and childbirth education. As Coordinator of Parent Education at Harrisburg Hospital, Joyce has presented her childbirth and parenting programs to over 5,000 expectant parents and planned and conducted seminars on family centered maternity care. Before joining Harrisburg Hospital in 1974, she taught eight years as a childbirth educator for a group of obstetricians and was an instructor of Obstetric Nursing at the Harrisburg Hospital School of Nursing.

Joyce is recognized as a Certified Childbirth Educator by Harrisburg Hospital having completed the criteria for childbirth educators recommended by the International Childbirth Education Association (ICEA), including the completion of ICEA Recognized Teacher Training and Teacher Enrichment Workshops. She is a member of ICEA, the Nurses Association of the American College of Obstetricians and Gynecologists (NAACOG) and serves on the advisory board for the Harrisburg Chapter March of Dimes.

Joyce is a graduate of Lancaster General Hospital School of Nursing, Lancaster, Pennsylvania and Millersville State College, Millersville, Pennsylvania and maintains membership on the Alumni Association of both institutions. In addition to her administrative and teaching responsibilities, she is a featured speaker at colleges, schools and outside organizations. Ms. Kieffer lives with her husband and two daughters in New Cumberland, Pennsylvania.

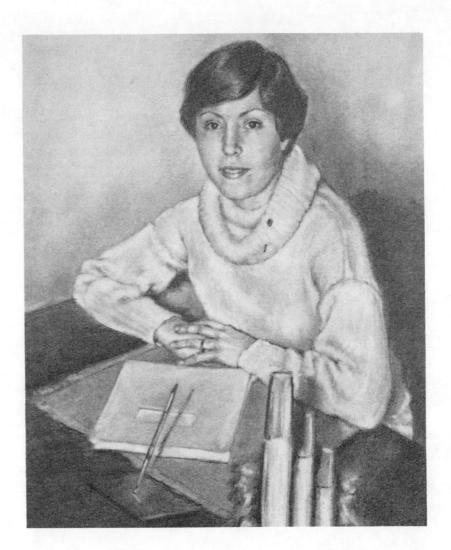

PREFACE

The beginnings of this manual really took place in 1966 when I was pregnant and ready to "retire" from my career in nursing education. A local obstetrician approached me about developing a prenatal class for his patients in their first pregnancy. Just having read *Thank You, Dr. Lamaze,* not only was I eager to teach prepared childbirth, I was naive enough to think I could be the test case.

There was very little information available to me as a childbirth educator or a mother-to-be. No breathing or relaxation guides, no literature—there was no proven support for my wish to have my husband with me during the birth of our baby. So I had very little to go on except a deep, personal commitment to change all that if I ever had the chance to do so.

Meanwhile, our daughter was born following a long labor with no husband present to share those hours and her arrival. Eighteen months later our second daughter was born. This time my husband stayed with me during labor but was turned away when I was taken to the delivery room. In neither experience was I able to touch or hold my baby until all the procedures for identification, weighing, eye treatment, etc., were completed. Nor was I allowed to unwrap or touch their naked bodies.

My husband touched them only once in the hospital. For a brief moment he felt the wonderful closing of the baby's hand over his little finger. So, we were almost strangers by the time we went home five days later.

My experiences were not unique or shocking in 1966. But the effect they had on me was profound. I knew there had to be a better way of preparing for childbirth and the beginning of parenthood.

As I gained experience as an educator, nurse, and parent, I began to write my own materials. When I was asked to be coordinator of parent education at a large urban teaching hospital, I eagerly accepted. By then my girls were in school, and I had eight years of experience in childbirth preparedness training in a private medical practice to my credit.

As I worked with people of all ages, races, nationalities and social backgrounds, I saw the need to provide more written information, including an easy-to-read but complete source of information on prepared childbirth that could be used for a variety of expectant parent education programs.

Therefore, this manual does not endorse any particular style or method of childbirth. The format is clear and complete and includes content which will help new parents through the early months. The individual teacher can incorporate his or her own style into the program. Certain sections of the manual can be assigned as outside reading and not even be included in class content. Other parts can be used as direct procedure in class, such as the section on "Relaxation and Breathing Exercises."

My experience with several thousand persons from age twelve to mid-fifties from the rich mixture of races and nationalities found in a large city has provided fertile ground for writing this manual for parents. Because of this spectrum of individual differences, I have taken great care to include information for the single as well as the married parent. I have also used the comments from hundreds of questionnaires in the sections on pregnancy, early parenting and their attendant emotional crises.

This manual was written to inform but not to manipulate, to help you understand the physical and emotional aspects of childbearing, but not to overwhelm. It can be read one section at a time, not following a particular sequence, or in its entirety from cover to cover. It is not meant to be a textbook or encyclopedia but an informative and enjoyable guide to prepare you for childbirth and early parenting.

TABLE OF CONTENTS

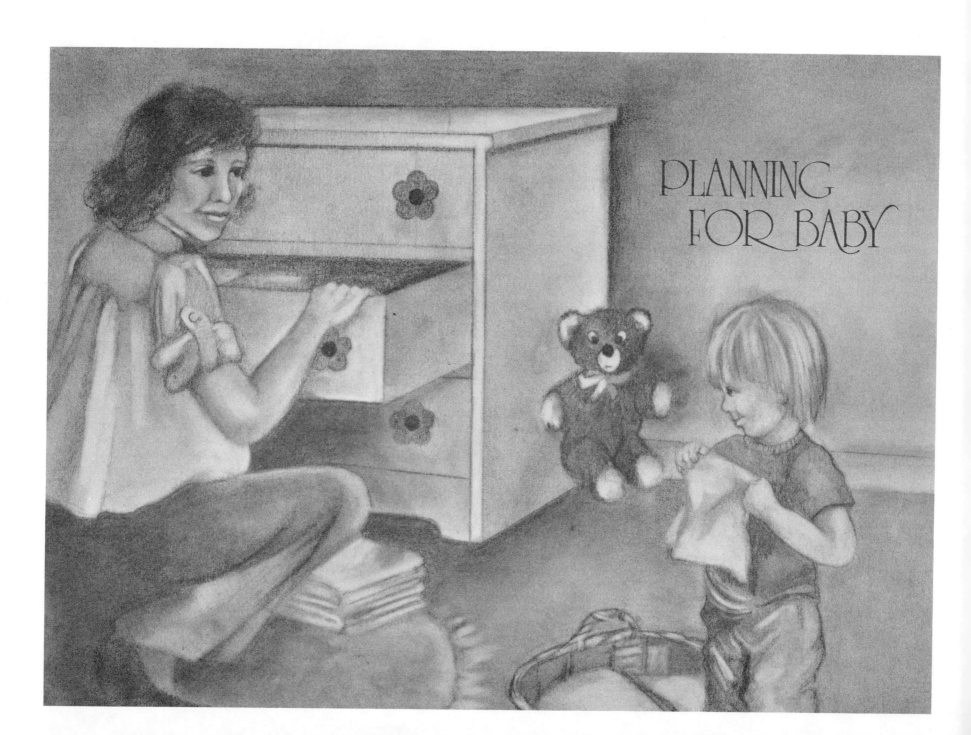

PLANNING FOR BABY

Part I: Planning for Baby

To Have . . . To Hold . . .

WHY "PREPARED" CHILDBIRTH?

Having a baby is a normal, natural process. It's a very challenging and intense physical and emotional experience. Like any event in a lifetime, things go smoothly if preparations are made ahead of time. Being prepared for childbirth takes away the mystery and fear.

Because of stories you have heard or movies you have seen, you may anticipate labor and birth to be painful and stressful. In real life, most birth experiences are very different from the movie versions of agony and suffering. It is true a woman may feel helpless and frightened during labor if she is unaware of what is happening to her body and doesn't know how to cope with it. The labor partner who is unprepared will see her suffering and feel helpless in trying to comfort her.

Fear of the unknown, loss of control and increased body tension during childbirth can exaggerate the pain. The "fear-tension-pain" cycle influences the muscular activity of the birth process, inhibits labor and intensifies discomfort.

By preparing for childbirth, you will not only learn what is going to happen during labor and birth, but also how to work constructively to advance the process. Instead of tensing with each contraction, you will consciously relax. You will also concentrate on a specific breathing pattern to maintain a proper oxygen level in your system. Your labor partner will not merely observe or cheer you on but will be an equal participant, giving you vital physical and emotional support.

Labor is hard work. However, knowing how to cooperate with the natural processes will make it easier for you.

TAKE CARE OF YOURSELF FOR BABY'S SAKE

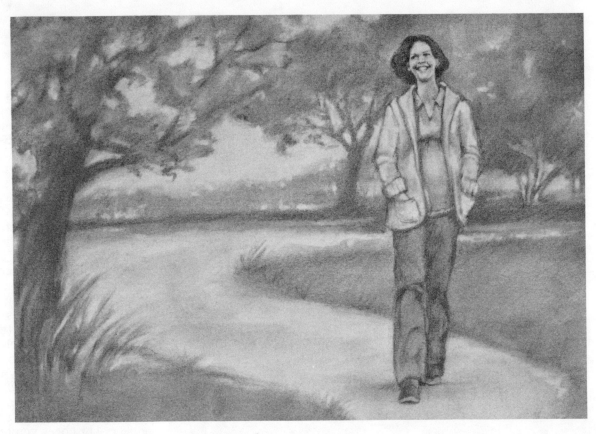

Every woman wants her baby to be born healthy. The best way to give your baby the gift of good health is to remain healthy yourself.

If you have just found out you're pregnant, you have the advantage of being able to protect your baby from harmful substances during the time growth and development is most rapid. This is the time when your baby's organs and tissues are most vulnerable to X-ray, viruses and drugs.

Even after your baby has passed the critical growth period of about 14 weeks gestation, what you eat and do still profoundly influence the health of your baby. It may be easier to think of your baby as a reality now that you are beginning to "show" and can feel the baby move. Do you know that your baby will gain all but about 1/2 pound of its birthweight in the last half of your pregnancy?

You can protect the health of your baby—up until the moment of birth. And you'll feel good about yourself knowing that you gave your baby the best possible start in life. Here are the steps you should take during your pregnancy to take good care of yourself and your unborn baby.

STEP 1:   GET GOOD MEDICAL CARE DURING YOUR PREGNANCY

Your baby's growth is very rapid early in pregnancy. Go to your family doctor, obstetrician, hospital maternity clinic or nurse midwife as soon as you suspect you are pregnant. That way if any problems do exist, they can be recognized and treated immediately. For example, you should notify your doctor or midwife

4

if any of the following signs appear:
- sharp or continuous abdominal pain
- bleeding from your vagina
- severe or continuous nausea and vomiting
- continuous or severe headaches
- swelling of face or hands or unusual swelling of feet or ankles
- decrease in fetal movement
- blurring of vision or spots before your eyes
- sudden increase in amount you urinate
- pain or burning when you urinate
- leakage of fluid from your vagina
- chills or fever

Follow the instructions they give you. If you don't understand or need more information or reassurance—ask! Poor prenatal care can result in premature birth or injury to both you and your baby.

STEP 2: EAT THE RIGHT FOODS

Try this mental exercise. Every time you eat, picture your baby eating the same thing. You certainly wouldn't feed your baby potato chips and cola for lunch.

It has been proven that good nutrition is probably the most important single factor affecting the health of unborn children. Impressive evidence also shows that good nutrition helps make labor easier and lowers the rate of toxemia, prematurity and stillbirth. And you'll feel better since eating a proper diet can prevent nausea, heartburn and constipation as well as reducing leg cramping and swelling.

If you are a teenage mother, you'll need to be even more careful about eating the right foods. Your body, especially your bones and teeth, are still growing right along with your unborn baby. Overweight, vegetarian and diabetic mothers need special nutritional counseling to meet their individual needs. If you are an expectant mother with special needs such as these, ask for help. It's important!

If you don't need special nutritional counseling during your pregnancy, here are some things you should know:

1. Gain between 24-27 pounds during your pregnancy.
2. Eat high quality protein foods, such as meat, fish, poultry, milk and eggs each day.
3. Take in a minimum of 2,100 calories to utilize protein properly.
4. Eat a balanced and varied diet that contains foods from each food group.
5. Choose foods with natural vitamins and minerals, such as whole grain breads, cereal, flour and rice, rather than highly refined sweets and starches.
6. Limit your intake of artificial sweetener preservatives and caffine; read labels before you buy.
7. Apply for food stamps or food vouchers provided by WIC (Women, Infants and Children) program if your income is limited.

The following list of foods should be included in your daily diet.

Milk—1 quart	provides protein and calcium
Eggs—1 or 2	is good source of protein and iron
Meats—6-8 oz.	provides protein, iron and B vitamins
Vegetables 3-4 serv.	include 1 dark green or dark yellow for A, E, C and B vitamins
Fruits—2 servings	include 1 citrus for vitamin C
Bread—3 servings Cereals	provides iron (whole grain), roughage, and vitamins
Water—3-4 glasses	prevents constipation

It doesn't matter if you eat three large meals, six small ones or a combination of meals and snacks. As long as your food is nutritious and you eat the right combination and amounts of food, you can eat whenever you feel hungry.

No matter what stage of pregnancy you are in—beginning, middle or end—it's never too soon or too late to start good eating habits. Your whole family will be healthier. And most of all, you'll have a more comfortable and enjoyable pregnancy, give birth to a healthier baby and be ready with a good supply of milk if you choose to breastfeed.

STEP 3: PROTECT YOURSELF WITH IMMUNIZATIONS

Try very hard to stay away from persons who are ill while you are pregnant. Avoid exposing yourself to someone with German measles (also known as rubella or 3-day measles). In the first three months of pregnancy, your baby can be seriously damaged by the rubella virus.

Immunity testing is available if you can't remember whether you had German measles. If you are susceptible, you can be vaccinated right after your baby is born to protect any future babies you may have. While you are at it, make sure your baby and older children are properly immunized, too.

STEP 4: BEWARE OF RADIATION

During pregnancy, the baby can be damaged if exposed to x-ray or radiation. Take special precautions during pregnancy. Have no X-rays taken without your doctor or dentist's full knowledge of your pregnancy or suspected pregnancy.

STEP 5: STOP SMOKING

Every time you inhale cigarette smoke you fill your lungs with nicotine, carbon monoxide and other harmful gases. Your blood carries these impurities through the umbilical cord into your baby's bloodstream. Smoking can restrict the baby's normal growth in the uterus. It can make your child underdeveloped and underweight at birth and prone to illness in the first critical weeks of life. New evidence also links cigarette smoking to crib death, spontaneous abortion, stillbirths, placenta previa and abnormally large areas of dead tissue on the placenta.

STEP 6: AVOID TAKING DRUGS

Many medications can cause birth defects when taken alone or combined with other drugs. Check with your doctor about the safety of taking drugs that may have been prescribed for you before your pregnancy began. Even common, over-the-counter drugs such as aspirin or decongestants can be harmful and should be used with permission by your doctor. Scientific re-search indicates that use of LSD, speed and other "street drugs" can cause extensive damage to an unborn child, resulting in mental retardation and gross physical defects.

Recently, drugs containing caffeine, as well as coffee, tea, cola drinks and chocolate, have been added to the list of potentially harmful substances. The Food and Drug Administration advises expectant mothers to abstain from products or drugs containing caffeine, or at least to practice moderation in their use.

STEP 7: ALCOHOL AND PREGNANCY DON'T MIX

If a pregnant woman has a drink, her unborn baby has a drink, too. Alcohol, like other things you eat and drink, passes through the placenta. It is believed that alcohol affects the baby's fast growing tissues, either killing cells or slowing their growth. Since the brain develops all through pregnancy, it stands to reason that this organ would be most affected by maternal drinking. If a woman drinks heavily while pregnant, her child may have a pattern of physical and mental birth defects, such as a small head and brain, mental deficiency, low IQ which does not improve with age, facial features with narrow eyes and low nasal bridges with short upturned noses. Almost half of these "fetal alcohol syndrome" babies have heart defects. The real tragedy of these defects is that they are completely preventable. The March of Dimes recommends, "If you're pregnant, don't drink. If you drink heavily, don't become pregnant."

STEP 8: BE AN INFORMED HEALTH CONSUMER

Seek information from your physician, nurse, midwife or child-birth educator concerning your care during pregnancy, childbirth and afterwards. Discuss alternatives, benefits, risks and expected results of treatments, procedures, drugs, etc. so that you can be a "partner" in your own and your baby's health care. Read about what you can do during your pregnancy to take good care of yourself. The National Foundation of March of Dimes prints two excellent booklets *Be Good To Your Baby Before It is Born* and *DATA: Drugs, Alcohol and Tobacco Abuse During Pregnancy*. Attend programs in preparation for childbirth and parenting to increase your knowledge and understanding. Remember, it's what you don't know that can hurt you or your unborn child.

BODY BUILDING EXERCISES

Taking care of yourself during pregnancy also includes readying your body for some hard work. The following exercises will help strengthen the muscles you will use in childbirth: squatting, tailor sitting, Kegel's and pelvic rocking. They are simple to learn and can be incorporated into almost any lifestyle. Just remember, start gradually and build up. If you feel tired or strained, stop. You can always resume later.

Exercising early in pregnancy will not only make you feel better, but can lessen any discomforts you may feel, such as backache and leg cramping.

If you practice these exercises faithfully each day, your muscle tone will be strong and firm. The specific areas of your body that need strengthening are the upper thighs, abdomen and pelvic floor. These muscles will be used and strained during the last stage of your labor when bearing down.

Wear comfortable clothes when doing these exercises, preferably a fabric that stretches. It could be embarrassing to split a seam or have a zipper come down.

SQUATTING

Get down in a squatting position and let your knees fall far apart. Hold onto something sturdy—you may have a tendency to fall forward. Practice this while doing any activity requiring you to bend your back. For example, squat down everytime you're putting clothes into a low dresser drawer or wiping up a spill from the floor. Get into a squatting position when you are preparing to lift a child or an object off the floor. Lift by straightening your legs rather than bending your back.

TAILOR SITTING

Sit on the floor with your legs drawn close to your body and ankles flat on the floor. If you are able to do so, place the soles of your feet together for further stretching and strengthening of the pelvic and thigh muscles. Assume this position while watching T.V., reading, sewing or just relaxing. Tailor sitting is much more comfortable than sitting in an overstuffed chair and not nearly as difficult to get out of. This position may also be used during labor, especially if discomfort is felt in the back.

A variation of this exercise is called the *"tailor press."* Place the soles of your feet together and pull them toward your body with your hands. This exercise also tones and stretches the pelvic floor and thigh muscles.

KEGEL'S EXERCISES (Pelvic Floor Exercises)

This exercise can be practiced during pregnancy but is most beneficial following birth. The muscles surrounding the vagina, urinary opening (urethra) and rectum will be used hard during birth. The area between the vagina and the rectum (perineum) is particularly stretched during birth and may be incised. (See *episiotomy* page 74)

Kegel's exercises are very beneficial in healing the pelvic floor, restoring its tone and circulation and minimizing the discomfort associated with the episiotomy.

During this exercise, all these muscles are gradually pulled upwards, as though you were stopping urination. Pull inward slowly to the count of ten; hold it several seconds and gradually release or relax to the count of ten.

Kegel's exercises can be done anytime, anywhere. Some women do Kegel exercises every time they are engaged in a particular activity, such as washing dishes or while waiting in line at the grocery store. Make good use of that time by doing some Kegel exercises. No one will even know you are doing it!

You may resume this exercise immediately following birth. Practice it several times each day for the next several months. Kegel's exercises can also be included in your daily exercise program for the rest of your life.

PELVIC ROCKING

This exercise may be done standing, lying flat on the floor with a pillow under your head and knees bent, or on all fours in a hands and knees position.

First tilt your pelvic girdle forward and out, so that the arch of the back is exaggerated. Then tuck the buttock muscles inward and tighten the abdominal muscles as though you were trying to tuck an imaginary tail between your legs. This motion tilts the pelvic girdle so that your back is flat against the floor or wall and there is no arch or space. Repeat this rocking motion ten times several times a day to relieve backache commonly experienced in the latter part of pregnancy.

ARM/SHOULDER ROTATIONS

Keeping your torso upright, hold your arms straight out at your sides. Slowly rotate first the right arm and then the left arm in a circular motion. Circle 10 times. This exercise increases shoulder flexibility, firms upper arms, and tones shoulder, upper back and chest muscles.

ELBOW/KNEE ROLL-UPS

Lie on your back on a carpeted floor. Bend your knees and place both feet flat on the floor. Clasp your fingers behind your neck. Inhale. As you exhale, slowly roll your upper body off the floor and raise your bent right leg toward your chest. Touch your left elbow to your right knee. Hold this position for several seconds and slowly return to starting position as you inhale. Repeat using your opposite knee and elbow. Do this exercise five to ten times a day to strengthen abdominal and thigh muscles.

BODY ROLL-UPS

Lie on your back on a carpeted floor. Bend your knees and place your feet flat on the floor, slightly apart. Let your hands rest on your thighs. Inhale. As you exhale, tuck your chin to your chest and roll both shoulders off the floor while you slowly slide your hands toward your knee. Hold your hands as close to your knees as you can without lifting your waistline off the floor. Hold that position, breathing normally, as you slowly count to 10. Slowly roll back to starting position. Repeat this exercise five to ten times a day.

Roll-ups are good for strengthening and firming abdominal muscles without straining your back.

LATERAL STRETCH

Stand upright using good posture with feet apart for balance. Bring your right arm up and over your head, stretching toward the left. Keep your left arm diagonally across your body at your waistline. Stretch that right arm up as far as possible—you should feel your ribs lifting and your waistline stretching. Keep your shoulders flat as though they were against the wall. Then slowly return to your starting position. Repeat five to ten times alternating arms.

This exercise is a great torso trimmer. It works your lateral abdominal and back muscles that form your waistline.

LEG SWINGS

Sit on a carpeted floor with your legs apart and straight out in front of you. Lean back on your hands placed about 12 inches from your buttocks. Lift your left leg and swing it all the way over to the right side of your body and touch your foot to the ground. Lift it up again, swing it back across your body to its original position. Now do the same thing with your right leg. Continue leg swings for several minutes.

Leg swings are super thigh firmers and they help strengthen front lateral abdominal muscles as well.

GROWTH & DEVELOPMENT OF YOUR UNBORN BABY

The month-to-month development of your baby will be much more meaningful, now that you know the steps to take to keep yourself and your baby healthy. The following chart outlines the growth of the fetus. Notice the tremendous increase in weight—upon reaching the fifth month, the fetus weighs 8 ounces and increases to a weight of seven to nine pounds at full term.

Don't hesitate to ask your physician questions about the development and size of your baby. Listen to the baby's heartbeat with a stethoscope or electronic device such as a "doptone" or a fetal monitor. Find out what position the baby is in and whether you can identify a foot or elbow where you feel the most kicking.

What a joy to think of your unborn child as a real and separate being as well as a part of yourself! Unborn babies have periods of rest and activity; they hiccough and suck their thumbs; they drink small amounts of amniotic fluid and excrete urine back into the fluid. Waste material forms in the bowel but is not normally passed until after birth. Both urine and bowel matter are odorless and bacteria free since the unborn child grows and develops in an environment which is sterile as long as the membranes remain unbroken.

There is no nerve connection between mother and baby, just two arteries and a vein where nutrients and wastes are exchanged, so a frightening experience or injury to the mother cannot result in a birthmark as old wives' tales may claim.

AGE	DEVELOPMENTAL CHARACTERISTICS
1 month (4 wks.)	¼ inch long. Backbone is apparent but is bent upon itself. The beginning of eyes, ears and nose make their appearance. Bulge on front of chest is early heart which is already pulsating and propelling blood through microscopic arteries. Buds are present as arms and legs.
2 months (8 wks.)	Has human face, arms, legs, fingers, toes, elbows and knees. Measures 1 inch, weighs 1/30 of an ounce. Has external genitalia, but not distinguishable. Head still very large as brain develops.
3 months (12 wks.)	Now measures over 3 inches and weighs almost 1 ounce. Sex is distinguishable. Fingers and toes become differentiated; finger and toe nails appear as fine membranes. Buds for all "baby" teeth are present. Primitive kidneys secrete small amounts of urine into the bladder. Fetus moves.
4 months (16 wks.)	Fetus grows to 4 ounces and approximately 6½ inches long. Sex definitely apparent.
5 months (20 wks.)	Has increased weight to 8 ounces and length to 10 inches. A fine downy hair called lanugo grows on the skin over the whole body. Baby's movements may be felt by the mother for the first time, referred to as "quickening." Physician may hear the baby's heart rate for the first time.
6 months (24 wks.)	The fetus now weighs 1½ pounds and measures 12 inches. It now looks like a baby, with the exception of the skin which is very thin and wrinkled. At this time, the skin develops fatty, cheesy substance called vernix to protect it. The fetus can survive at this size but chances are still slim.
7 months (28 wks.)	Measuring 15 inches and weighing 2½ pounds, the fetus has a chance of surviving if born.

AGE	DEVELOPMENTAL CHARACTERISTICS
8 months (32 wks.)	The fetus measures 16½ inches and weighs about 4 pounds. Weight gain and growth is rapid. Vernix and lanugo still present and protecting skin.
9 months (36 wks.)	Fetus is now quite mature, but at 6 pounds and 18 inches may have some growing to do. Gains ½ pound a week at this time.
10 months (38-40 wks.)	Mature and has firm fingernails that protrude beyond end of fingers. Most lanugo is gone but vernix remains thick. Weighs 7 to 9 pounds and measures 18 to 22 inches.

The length of pregnancy varies greatly. It may range from 240 to 300 days and be normal. The average duration from conception is 9½ lunar months (38 weeks or 266 days). If counting from the first day of the last menstrual period it is 10 lunar months (40 weeks or 280 days).

If you are interested in learning more about the development of your unborn baby, an excellent book with award-winning photographs is *A Child Is Born* by Lennert Nilson. A second book, *The Child Before Birth* by Linda Annis also includes the effects of external environmental influences on the unborn child.

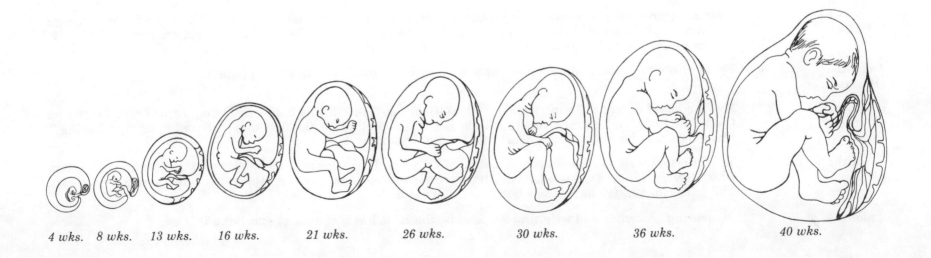

4 wks.   *8 wks.*   *13 wks.*   *16 wks.*   *21 wks.*   *26 wks.*   *30 wks.*   *36 wks.*   *40 wks.*

To Have . . . To Hold . . .

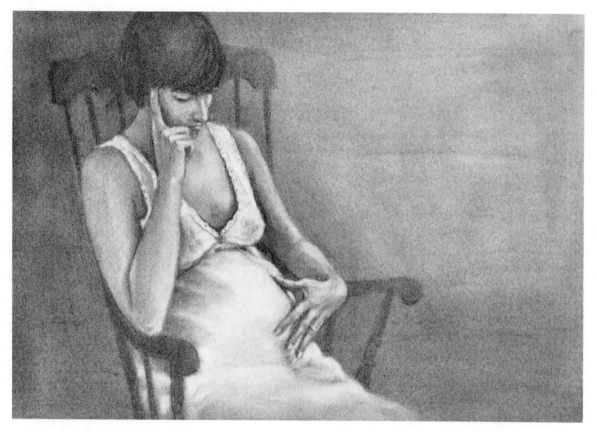

THE EMOTIONS OF PREGNANCY

Human pregnancy is a biological event and an unforgettable emotional experience.

We often have feelings about things that happen to us. They are part of our natural being, like breathing and sleeping, and can be an asset or a liability depending on how well we cope with them.

Each person handles the stress of becoming a parent in his or her own way. A number of factors can influence this, such as, previous experiences in coping with change or preconceived notions about pregnancy and parenting. Being able to rely on a person whose care and support you can count on may help make this adjustment easier.

If you are married, this support person is probably your spouse. Sometimes circumstances compel the expectant mother to find a substitute. If you are a single parent, you may still want the baby's father to be part of the birth experience to help forge an alliance which can strengthen you both.

A mother on her own finds herself most vulnerable of all. She needs a friend, a relative or possibly another single mother to become that support person during her pregnancy and childbirth. Many hospitals encourage single mothers to attend prepared childbirth classes and permit a labor partner or companion to accompany her during labor and birth.

The following questions may help you to be more aware of your own feelings and to be more sensitive to the feelings of your partner. You will find that other expectant parents have similar feelings that quite often are not openly discussed. For example, complete these sentences in your own words:

1. My biggest fear about this pregnancy is:

2. I would feel better during this pregnancy if my partner would:

3. What worries me most about this child coming into my life is:

4. The thing I would like my partner to understand most during this pregnancy is:

5. I'd like to be able to talk to my partner about:

6. After the birth, I am most concerned about:

If you exchange answers with your partner, you will understand and appreciate the other's feelings about this pregnancy. It may even help to talk to one of your friends who is expecting a baby or has small children. Be reassured that others have many of the same feelings and experiences.

NEWBORN BABY'S LAYETTE

Expectant mothers have a pressing need to get ready for the baby, sometimes far ahead of the time the expectant father feels it is necessary. It compares to the "nesting instinct" found in other mammals.

Perhaps by preparing the room and shopping for some baby clothes, the pregnant woman feels she has fulfilled a mission. In instances where labor and birth are premature and the "preparation of the nest" has not been completed, the new mother often frets and feels unsettled until it has been accomplished.

Men are sometimes perplexed by this urge, but they would be wise to recognize its importance and go along with the preparations and shopping.

Consider these suggestions when purchasing items for a layette: safety, launderability, ease of application and economy.

The following items are necessary for the care of a newborn infant through the first six months of age. They should be of a high quality so that they retain their fit through repeated washings, should be easy to put on and take off and should not contain wool or be fastened with large buttons or a drawstring around the neck. The quantity of each item is sufficient if laundered two or three times a week.

6 undershirts—6 month size, short sleeves, snap closing

8 sleepers, crawlers or kimonos

3 to 4 dozen diapers—plus 1 dozen disposable for emergency use

3 receiving blankets

1 sweater set (sweater, cap and booties)

1 heavy crib blanket or bunting

6 bibs

2 large bath towels, 6 washcloths

3 crib sheets

1 mattress cover or large pad

3 waterproof lap pads

8 waterproof panties.

The following items are nice to have, but are not absolutely necessary. Many times they are received as gifts:

shawl to wear over clothing and cotton blankets.

dresses, suits, soft shoes, socks

extra sleepers, undershirts

second sweater set

snow suit or heavy knitted jacket and pants set

NURSERY FURNITURE & EQUIPMENT

When purchasing items for use in the baby's room, consider safety, economy and size of the room.

A baby does not need much furniture during the first few months of life. As long as the items used are in good repair and are painted with lead free (non-toxic) paint, they can be borrowed, purchased or constructed at home.

The following items are essential for the care and comfort of a newborn infant during the first six months of age:

crib**—bassinet* can be used for a short time (3 months) or a clothes basket or deep dresser drawer.

firm mattress—a folded blanket protected by a heavy plastic or rubber mattress cover and pillow case should be used for a mattress in a bassinet, never a bed pillow.

a bureau or chest of drawers

sturdy flat surface for bathing and changing baby—can be a card table, bathinette, or a regular nursery dressing stand.

infant seat—should be very sturdy so that an active baby cannot easily tip it over; can be used as a feeding chair, and enables the baby to look around and be carried about.

crib bumper—to prevent baby's head and extremities from going through crib slats.

vaporizer—indispensable for use in helping baby to breathe during colds and other illnesses. The cold mist type is usually recommended over a steam vaporizer because it is safer and more effective.

car seat**—choose one that is recommended by the U.S. Consumer Product Safety Commission and follow manufacturer's directions for proper use.

tray containing:

thermometer
vasoline
mild, unscented bath soap
cotton balls
cotton-tipped applicators
rubbing alcohol
safety pins stuck in cake of soap wrapped with adhesive tape
fine-toothed comb or brush
baby powder or lotion if desired—check with physician before using
fingernail scissors

The following items are also nice to have as baby grows older:

playpen with pad (and bumper if wooden playpen is used)
highchair
stroller or carriage
rocking chair (adult)—considered essential by many mothers
mobile (brightly colored animals or birds hung on crib to amuse baby)
baby tub or foam "tubby"

**More about your baby's crib:*

The following safety checklist is recommended to prevent accidents from unsafe sleeping conditions. If you can answer yes to any of these questions, you need to make the necessary corrections before you can consider your baby safe from crib accidents.

A. Mattress
   1. Size. Is there a space greater than 2.5 cm (1 inch) between the mattress and the crib sides or ends?
   2. Support. Does the mattress sag in any spot when the baby lies on it? (Check both the middle and the edges.) Can the plastic mattress cover be removed?

B. Crib Sides and Ends
   1. Are there any splits, cracks, toe holds or old paint visible?
   2. Can the rails be pulled out, away from the side of the crib?
   3. Are the spaces between the slats more than 6 cm (2 3/8 inches)?

4. Can the rails fall down accidentally? (Shake them and apply pressure to the top.)
5. When the mattress is in the lowest position and the rails are up, is there less than a 66 cm (26 inches) difference between the two?

C. Accessories

Are there any string-like objects in the crib, used either as toys or for repairs? Is there a cradle gym, a pacifier around the child's neck, or medals on chains?

D. Position

Is the crib positioned beside any other furniture, such as a chair, bureau, radiator or another bed, that the baby could use to climb out?

Recommendations for Care of Infant in Crib:

1. Never leave the infant alone when the side rails are down.

2. Lower the mattress before the baby can sit unassisted and set it at the lowest position as soon as the infant can stand.

3. Leave no toys or other articles in the crib that can be used as steps for climbing out.

4. Do not hang crib toys within reach of the infant.

5. No longer use the crib when the height of the side rails is less than three fourths of the child's height.

6. Position the crib away from windows and other furniture that could be used to climb out.

7. Position crib away from radiators or portable heaters.

**More about your baby's car seat:*

Car seats hold precious cargo. Always be sure to use one for your baby, starting with the first trip home from the hospital. Make sure you select a car seat that is approved by ACTS (Action for Child Transportation Safety) and use it according to directions.

In some communities the American Automobile Association will lend or rent approved infant, toddler and older child car seats to members and non-members alike.

Holding a baby or child on your lap or using an old car seat that only hooks under or over the passenger seat is not safe. Your baby needs to be properly protected. Use a safe car seat that can be held in place by an adult seat belt.

And while you're at it, you can buckle up too. Authorities suggest that you wear a seat belt while you're pregnant. Research has shown that the most serious risk to your unborn baby is that you may be injured. Sit tall and place the lap belt as low as possible on your hips under the baby. For added protection, wear the shoulder harness too.

PREPARING SIBLINGS FOR NEW BABY

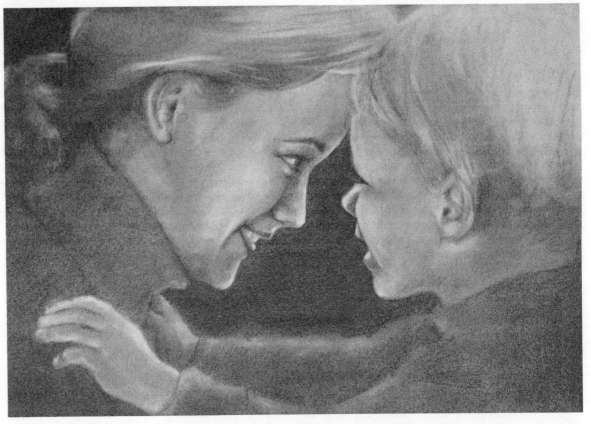

Most parents are concerned about how an older child or children will react to a new baby in the family. Parents are concerned they won't have enough time or patience for another child.

Much of what you do about preparing an older child for a new sibling and coping with any conflicts that arise later is dependent on your nature and your relationship with that child. If you are generally patient and understanding of the normal behavior and development of your child at his/her age, your expectations will probably be realistic. A child who has a trusting relationship with his/her parents will probably be less threatened by a new baby than a child whose own needs are not being met most of the time. It may be worth spending some additional time with your child before the baby is born. Then continue sharing special times to-

gether as often as possible after the new baby arrives.

The age difference between the older child and the new baby will also help to determine appropriate ways to talk to your child and ease his/her adjustment. But regardless of your child's age, preparation for a new baby should begin when you feel comfortable talking about your pregnancy and when you are reasonably sure that your son or daughter will benefit from knowing about it at that particular time.

For example, even small children are aware that "mommy's getting fat" and notice you're spending time getting the house and nursery ready for the baby.

Some parents make the mistake of confusing their children by misinforming them. Telling a child that the baby comes out of the "bellybutton" or that mommy goes to the hospital to pick up the baby is not only confusing, but he or she may later mistrust you for not telling the truth. A simple explanation using the correct terms in a matter-of-fact tone, provides them with accurate information and sets the stage for healthy attitudes about human reproduction. Contrary to what you may think, children rarely find these things disgusting or upsetting.

Let your child or children touch your abdomen and feel the baby move. Tell them how it felt when he or she was inside you. Ask your doctor or nurse to let your child listen to the baby's heartbeat. Many physicians welcome children during prenatal visits and will help you prepare them for the new baby. And, a small, but growing number of hospitals and birth centers allow children to be present during the birth.

Another way to help a child prepare for the change and separation is by allowing the child to spend a few days or a night away from home before the baby is born. Be honest and clear about the fact that you will be going to the hospital for a few days and will be coming home again. Perhaps your children may visit you in the hospital. A story book about "where babies come from" and a visit to a new baby's house can be very reassuring, especially to a young child.

Ask your child "How do you feel about having a new baby brother or sister?" Allow your child to be honest about feelings, realizing that it is perfectly normal and natural for an older child to have mixed feelings or even dislike the idea of having a new baby in the family. Accept the idea that your child may not be enthusiastic about the baby and perhaps confused about how it will look and behave. Reassure your child that you understand why he or she may not want to share Mommy and Daddy with a baby, but that "We're sure there is enough of us to go around!"

This approach is more healthful than forcing a child to feel love for a new sibling or refusing to allow the child to talk about negative feelings. At the same time, you can let your child know that he or she will not be allowed to hurt the baby. If an older child is encouraged to help with the baby, the feeling of being "left-out of the family" will be lessened.

If your child is between one and three, he or she will still need a good deal of physical care, such as weaning and toilet training. Children at this age are not independent and feel especially threatened by the birth of a sibling. Parents may still regard the young child as their "baby" and may have difficulty letting go. On the other hand, parents are bewildered when the child becomes defiant over efforts to wean him from dependency. It's quite normal for children at this age to be negative and defiant; and if there is a new baby in the family, the child finds it easy to behave this way because a new brother or sister has moved into his or her "territory."

Children three to five are probably able to play outside the home and may even attend a nursery or church school or perhaps a play group. This helps them establish a sense of independence and acceptance. A child this age is also better able to reason and be reasoned with. Of course, time spent with parents is still highly valuable and important!

What children of all ages really want and need most is to feel special and loved. Parents convey these warm feelings by spending time and doing things with their children. Even short periods of one-to-one play times, times when children have your undivided attention are very effective. They help you say to your children "you are very special."

Sometimes this may mean letting the dishes go or mowing the lawn later. Fathers can be especially close to an older child by assuming some of the caretaking jobs for that child or spending time together going on errands and playing. If children feel they are getting enough attention, they seldom resort to negative behavior in order to get it. Children quickly learn how to get a response from their behavior, and a negative response is better than none at all.

Learn to trust yourselves as parents. You are the best judge of what is best for your children. Asking advice from other parents, your own parents, your physician or even reading a good book on parenting can all help; but all of these so-called "experts" can only recommend in general—your situation is uniquely yours and yours in particular. Follow your own instincts; use common sense and you'll almost never go wrong.

Forgetting your suitcase on the way to the hospital seems to be a standard joke among expectant parents. If you do forget to take it with you, that's okay. You probably won't need it until after the baby is born, and you are settled into your room. By this time someone can bring it in for you.

If you are only staying in the hospital or birthcenter for a short time, simply pack a tote bag.

The following items are usually necessary for a three to seven day hospital stay. For yourself:

slippers	going home clothes for you
bathrobe	(allow for extra size of bust and waist)
bras (3-4)	lightweight nightgown or pajamas (4-5)
sanitary belt	underpanties (5-7)
make-up	reading and writing material
toiletries	birth announcements
extra Kleenex	hair care equipment
	(shampoo, dryer, if permitted)

For baby's going home clothes:

undershirts	waterproof pants
diapers (2)	receiving blanket
diaper pins (2)	sweater, cap, and heavy blanket
nightgown	(if cool weather)

If you are planning to breastfeed your baby, remember to take these items:

nursing bras

button-down-the front nightgown

nursing pads if not provided by hospital
  (should not have plastic liners)

your copy of book on breastfeeding (optional)
  (See suggested reading list on page 79 for names and authors)

Many hospitals provide a maternity kit which contains approximately:

3 dozen hospital-size sanitary pads

4 disposable washcloths

2 plastic bed pads

1 sanitary belt

shower cap

To help you feel ultra-prepared, pack in a separate paper bag or tote bag a "labor kit" containing personal touches from home. You might enjoy your own bed pillow covered with a bright cheery pillow case. Your labor kit can be both fun and functional. Put this manual in your kit first, then add:

chap stick

food for labor partner (sandwich, apple, candy bar)

time passers (playing cards, book, magazine)

nice smelling talcum powder

kneesocks or sneaker socks

sour lollypops, lifesavers or chewing gum if permitted

sock with tennis ball to place behind small of back
  for relief from back labor

focal points (pictures, decals, etc.)

Check off items not provided by your hospital. You may want to tear out this page for a handy shopping and packing list.

However, it is reassuring to pack your suitcase ahead of time, possibly during the last month or weeks of your pregnancy. Many mothers regard it as a visible sign that they are in control of things and ready to go at a moment's notice.

THINGS TO DO BEFORE THE DUE DATE

1. CHOOSE A FAMILY DOCTOR OR PEDIATRICIAN

Choose a pediatrician for your baby. If you already have a family doctor with whom you feel comfortable and confident, consider having him or her care for the baby also. A pediatrician may be advisable should your baby need more specialized care. Speak to the doctor before your baby is due to find out about hospital and office visits, feeding preferences, how calls to the doctor are handled (call time, answer service, etc.) and fees. You have time now to find a physician who best suits your needs and is most compatible to your ideas on child care and parenting.

2. DRUGSTORE

Locate a drugstore in your area which delivers and have the drugstore's telephone number handy when calling your pediatrician. You might also inquire if the store is open 24 hours. Do they deliver prescriptions only, or is there a minimum purchase policy in order to have things delivered? Many drugstores accept major credit cards, which is convenient.

3. YOUR WARDROBE FOLLOWING CHILDBIRTH

In the last few weeks of your pregnancy, wash and return your borrowed maternity clothes and sort out the loose fitting clothes you plan to wear following birth. Your waistline and bustline will be temporarily expanded. Wrap-around skirts and shifts are useful during this period.

If you are nursing, you will need button-down-the front clothing and nightgowns. Pull-up-from-the-waist tops (sweaters, shells or blouses) are the most convenient to wear when nursing away from your home. Several patterns use invisible zippers placed on convenient seamlines for nursing.

4. WAYS TO ORGANIZE

1. Get the baby equipment and furniture set up and ready to use.
2. Launder baby clothes and put into drawers. Laundering new items helps to remove excess lint and softens the fabric.
3. Think ahead to birthdays, holidays, anniversaries, etc., and buy gifts and cards now that you will need in the two months following birth. During the first few weeks at home, it will be difficult for you to find some free time to shop.
4. Think ahead to the next season and get the family's clothes ready now.
5. Write out detailed directions for other children during your hospitalization. Include their schedule of meals, naps, bedtime, school or carpools, usual snack foods, etc. It is also helpful to the parent substitute if you will include a list of the absolute "don'ts."

5. SAFETY CHECK YOUR HOME

While you have time before the baby arrives, make your home a safe place for children to live.

1. All medicines and chemicals should be in a locked cabinet.
2. Remove cleaning items from underneath sinks and place high out of reach or in a locked cabinet.
3. Block unused electrical outlets with dummy plugs.
4. An accident handbook is a wise investment which should be read now and placed in a handy location for easy reference.
5. Have emergency numbers permanently attached to telephones. These should include numbers for physicians (especially the pediatrician), fire and police departments, poison control center and your nearest neighbor, relative or friend.

Accidents often occur when children are hungry or tired, when parents are rushed or under emotional stress or when children are under the care of an unfamiliar person or in an unfamiliar location. Therefore, think ahead and take special precautions for these times.

6. PLAN IMMUNIZATIONS FOR YOUR BABY*

The childhood diseases that terrified your parents today seem as remote and harmless as the dinosaur. Worry disappeared when vaccines were developed. But no matter how effective a vaccine is, it can only work if a child receives it.

An estimated 40% of the children in America today are not receiving the vaccines they should, and thus, they remain unprotected against very preventable diseases. The people at your hospital haven't forgotten the deaths and permanent disabilities these illnesses caused before vaccines were developed. They want to be sure that your child receives all the protection available. And they'd like to see preventable diseases become extinct.

Make and keep the necessary appointments for immunizations. And if you have an older child at home, be sure that his or her immunizations are up to date, too. Give your child a good shot at health!

The American Academy of Pediatrics recommends the following schedule of immunizations:

AGE	IMMUNIZATION NEEDED
2 months	First Polio, First DPT (Diphtheria, Pertussis, Tetanus)
4 months	Second DPT, Second Polio
6 months	Third DPT
1 year	TB Test
15 months	Measles, Mumps, Rubella
18 months	Fourth DPT, Third Polio
4-6 years	DPT Booster, Polio Booster
14-16 years	Tetanus, Diphtheria

*Printed with permission from the American Hospital Association

7. THINK ABOUT BREAST OR BOTTLE FEEDING

The decision to breast or bottle feed should be made before your baby is born. It's a personal decision—only you can make it. You may be influenced by family and friends, but choose the method that you sincerely prefer rather than one others would like you to choose. If you choose to bottle feed your baby, you will need to purchase or borrow a disposable nurser set or sterilizer, bottles and nipples. There is no special preparation necessary. However, it may be a good idea to purchase only what you will need for the first few weeks after your baby is born. Your experience in feeding your baby will be the best indicator of whether or not that feeding system is satisfactory for you and your baby. More information about bottle feeding can be found on page 60.

If you decide to breast feed your baby, you should begin preparing your breasts in the final 6 to 8 weeks of your pregnancy. This will help to condition your nipples for breastfeeding and minimize the soreness some women experience in the early nursing period. The following simple procedures should be practiced daily, preferably when you are bathing and have clean hands:

1. Massage. Gently massage breasts with your hands or terry wash cloth, starting at your chest wall and working toward the nipple.

2. Expose the nipples. Going without a bra for part of the day or wearing nursing bras with the flaps down exposes the nipple and areola so that friction from clothing accustoms these areas to slight stress.

3. Nipple rolling. Gently grasp nipple at its base with thumb and forefinger. Pull nipple gently outward and roll back and forth. Continue pulling and rolling evenly around entire nipple.

Whether you plan to nurse your baby or not, the breasts should be well supported by a bra that covers the entire breast and has wide comfortable straps. It should have several rows of hooks to accomodate a change in size when your breasts enlarge during pregnancy and when engorgement takes place following birth.

If you notice colostrum leaking from your breasts during pregnancy or if you experience leakage of breast milk during the nursing period, a folded, ironed man's handkerchief is an ideal liner for your bra. The handkerchief is cleaner and less expensive than nursing pads you can purchase because it may be used over and over again. Bras and nursing pads with plastic liners should be avoided since they don't allow for adequate circulation of air around the nipple.

THE
NATURAL PROCESS
OF CHILDBIRTH

Part II: The Natural Process of Childbirth

A. Labor Guide
B. Relaxation and Breathing Exercises for Labor and Birth
C. Special Message for the Labor Partner
D. Cesarean Childbirth
E. Guide to Medications and Anesthetics Used During Childbirth
F. Commonly Used Diagnostic Tests
G. Emergency Childbirth

LABOR GUIDE

As you read earlier, labor is hard work but can be made much easier by knowing how to do the job. This labor guide is designed to familiarize you with the stages of labor and their characteristics, the emotional reactions commonly experienced during each stage and the appropriate comfort and support measures.

Read the entire labor guide and then come back to the first stage to review it in greater detail. Since the first stage of labor is the longest and involves many physical and emotional changes, it has been broken down into three phases—first, middle and transition. Breathing techniques vary, but they all require the mother and the labor partner to practice and become familiar with them.

Three breathing exercises are used: slow chest breathing, accelerated or rapid shallow chest breathing and pant-blow breathing. After you read the Relaxation and Breathing Guide on pages 30-35, come back to this Labor Guide and use it to "rehearse" your labor over and over through all phases and stages.

Labor varies from one woman to another. You may quickly pass through one phase into another; you also may not even recognize that you are in labor until you have passed completely through the early phases. Also, certain types of medications may influence the progress of your labor or your perception of it.

When you think you're in labor call your physician or midwife. Ask when you should start the trip to the hospital. As a rule, when your contractions are approximately six to eight minutes apart for a first baby and ten to twelve minutes apart for the second—it's time to go!

If you already have children and have a history of rapid labors, you will want to leave much earlier in your labor. And, of course, if your membranes rupture or you have any bright bleeding, call your physician or maternity clinic right away.

Possibly only a few of the breathing techniques outlined in this manual will be selected for use in your preparation for childbirth program. (See pages 32-35) If this is the case, practice those selected very carefully. It is not so much *which* particular pattern of breathing you use, but how familiar the mother, the partner, the physician and nurses are with those breathing patterns.

STAGE	CHARACTERIZED BY	EMOTIONAL REACTION	COACHING AND SUPPORT
First stage (Effacement and Dilatation) 0-4 cms.	CONTRACTIONS: Every 5-20 minutes lasting 30-45 seconds.* ●Mild & irregular, then becoming stronger and regular.* ●May be felt as menstrual cramps, gas, backache, pelvic pressure, or a tightening down low in the area of the pubic bone or groin area, top of legs. SHOW: Begins as a slightly pink mucous discharge.	Excited and relieved. Some apprehension. Sociable and talkative between contractions. Air of anticipation. Impatient and eager for progress. Labor may temporarily stop or regress after hospital admission due to over-excitement.	AVOID FATIGUE. DO NOT EAT. CALL PHYSICIAN IF MEMBRANES RUPTURE. Time frequency and duration of contractions. Go about doing normal activity: light house work, read, walking, play cards, etc. Call physician when contractions are 10 minutes apart for multips and 5 minutes apart for primips.

The Natural Process of Childbirth

STAGE	CHARACTERIZED BY	EMOTIONAL REACTION	COACHING AND SUPPORT
First stage (Cont.)	MEMBRANES: May rupture up to 24 hours before labor or any time during labor; they may also be ruptured by the doctor. After rupture, fluid may trickle or gush from vagina. May urinate frequently. May have loose bowels. Lightening (baby dropping) may occur in multi-paras.		Finish packing and if necessary, arrange for care of any other children. Labor partners: Give support and encouragement. Remind her to relax. If doctor or midwife agrees, encourage her to walk. This may help stimulate labor, and the time will pass more quickly. Start slow chest breathing when necessary to maintain relaxation, take cleansing breath after each contraction.
Middle phase of first stage 5-7 cms. Usually shorter than early phase.	CONTRACTIONS: Every 3-5 minutes lasting 45-60 seconds. •Businesslike, more regular, frequent and intense; building to a peak more rapidly. •Last longer and are more uncomfortable. SHOW: Heavier in amount and more blood tinged. May become nauseated and vomit—good sign labor is progressing. May experience increased discomfort in back. (Back labors occur in 25–30% of labors.) Are often due to baby's being in a face up or posterior position.	May appear tense and restless. Increasingly dependent and needs quiet companionship. Ill defined doubts, wonders if she can cope with contractions to come. Works hard during contractions and prefers not to talk or be distracted. May breathe too rapidly and deeply (hyperventilate) causing temporary panic-numbness of hands, tingling around mouth, twitching of legs. If this happens, cup hands over mouth and breath your own air or, hold your breath for a short period after the contraction is over.	Hospital admission: brief history, and physical exam. May have prep and enema (policies vary). Needs frequent encouragement, coaching, and companionship. Needs quiet calm environment. Accept her irritability and praise her efforts. Remind her to: urinate and change positions often; concentrate on one contraction at a time; rest completely between contractions. Offer cold washcloth, mouthwash, ice chips if permitted.

STAGE	CHARACTERIZED BY	EMOTIONAL REACTION	COACHING AND SUPPORT
Middle phase of first stage (Cont.)		Relaxation is difficult.	For back labor: Use back pressure with heel of hand, rolled towel, etc. Avoid lying on back. Rotate side-lying, tailor sitting, on all fours, kneeling positions. Apply heat or ice to her lower back. Begin using accelerated chest breathing sometimes referred to as "ha" breathing. Increase breathing rate only as a contraction builds. When contraction starts to subside, slow down rate of breathing accordingly.
Transition phase of first stage (effacement and dilatation.) 8-10 cms.	CONTRACTIONS: Every 1-2 minutes lasting 60-90 seconds; very strong and long, at its peak almost immediately and almost on top of each other (seem continuous to mother). SHOW: Heavy and dark. May have momentary nausea and vomiting; natural amnesia, leg cramps and trembling, backache. Face is flushed and perspired. May feel hot or cold, very restless. Relaxation is very difficult; feels sleepy between contractions.	Irritable, sensitive and short tempered, finds it difficult to talk. Overwhelmed and wants to give up; bewildered and temporarily discouraged. Has considerable difficulty concentrating and relaxing. May be surprised, overwhelmed or even frightened at the irresistible urge to push.	TRY NOT TO LEAVE HER ALONE. NEEDS CONSTANT ENCOURAGEMENT, COACHING AND REASSURANCE of normalcy of sensations and feelings. NEEDS FIRM, POSITIVE GUIDANCE; CONTINUOUS LOW KEY VERBAL COACHING and breathing with her through each contraction often helps.

STAGE	CHARACTERIZED BY	EMOTIONAL REACTION	COACHING AND SUPPORT
Transition phase of first stage (Cont.)			REMIND HER: •this phase is short and its completion means birth is near. •semi-sitting position with knees spread apart and heels together is helpful. •take one contraction at a time and conquer it. Use pant-blow breathing pattern. Take cleansing breath after each contraction.
Second Stage (expulsion) Pushing and birth.	CONTRACTIONS: Every 3–5 minutes lasting 60–75 seconds; powerful, expulsive in nature, but farther apart. Usually an irresistible urge to push. Pushing feels good if perineum is relaxed and you work with the urge to push. Rectal bulging, backache ceases. As head moves down birth canal, there may be a burning, splitting sensation as baby's head crowns the perineum. Perineum "irons out" and becomes white and thin. Episiotomy may be performed under local anesthesia.	Very tired but a revival of determination and burst of energy. Rectal pressure may cause anxiety and hesitation to push. Tremendous effort may produce distorted facial expressions and grunting sounds. Is usually drowsy and peaceful between contractions. Has self concern, indifferent to her surroundings, uninhibited, excited, impatient for progress. As birth draws near, excitement and mental alertness replaces drowsiness.	WORK WITH DOCTOR AND NURSE. Needs coaching with each contraction. May forget how to push. Suggest she push toward vagina and make full use of each contraction. Remind her to: •relax perineum •pant when doctor says to stop pushing •rest fully between contractions. Tell her when head is visible and praise her accomplishments.

STAGE	CHARACTERIZED BY	EMOTIONAL REACTION	COACHING AND SUPPORT
	Upon the doctor's order to stop pushing, baby is born between contractions, head first, then shoulders and rest of baby slips out easily.	Interest shifts to baby, its appearance and normalcy.	
Third Stage (placental) Separation and expulsion of placenta. Very brief stage, often unnoticed by mother.	CONTRACTIONS: Temporarily cease after birth. Uterus rises in abdomen and becomes globular in shape (size of grapefruit). Umbilical cord lengthens, indicating separation of placenta. Uterus contracts to expel placenta. Oxytocin injection may be given to contract uterus and reduce bleeding. Episiotomy repaired with local anesthetic.	Euphoria; pure ecstasy, relief, gratitude, disbelief, wonder, joy, may cry uncontrollably. Feels proud and fulfilled. Very hungry and tired, but too excited to really notice. May be annoyed when contractions resume. Delighted with flat abdomen. Often unaware of placental expulsion or episiotomy repair. Cools off in a hurry, may shake, teeth may chatter.	Rejoice with her over baby's birth. Reassure her of baby's normalcy. Touch and hold baby. Care of eyes, cord, etc. are normal procedures and can be done later or while baby is in mother's arms. If mother chooses to breast feed, put baby to the breast. Baby's sucking instinct is usually strong at birth. This early feeding will reinforce it and provide valuable stimulation for the production of breast milk. Praise her accomplishments. Sit down and enjoy your baby together. Warm blanket and a hot beverage feel good.

*To time contractions, you will need a watch or clock with a second hand. When a contraction begins, write down the exact time it began and the exact time it ended. This is called the duration of length of the contraction. When the next contraction begins, again note the exact time. The length of time between the beginning of the previous contraction and the beginning of the second contraction is how far apart they are occurring, or the frequency of the contractions.

For example:

Duration   Duration

Frequency   Frequency

RELAXATION & BREATHING EXERCISES FOR LABOR & BIRTH

The core of a preparation for childbirth program is learning the relaxation and breathing techniques. But learning how to relax without knowing how to keep your breathing in harmony with the contraction is like doing a job with a tool missing. In other words, learning breathing exercises without learning how to relax during a contraction is equally ineffective. Learn them both and you have the tools you need to make the job easier and safer.

This Relaxation and Breathing Exercises Guide is meant to be just that—a guide. The extent to which you use it and practice the techniques both in your classes and at home may vary. In almost all types of childbirth programs you will be encouraged to practice the exercises each day during the last six weeks of your pregnancy.

The first section deals with comfortable positions during labor. Practice relaxation and breathing exercises in every position so you feel comfortable with all of them. Two basic types of relaxation techniques are described next, followed by a detailed section on the breathing exercises. Before going on, carefully read the "four points to remember" preceding the actual exercises. This will help you form a healthful attitude about using breathing techniques during your labor.

The last section describes and outlines positions for pushing the baby down the birth canal. You can try the positions used in pushing but do not practice the actual bearing down unless you have obtained permission to do so. Some physicians feel vigorous practice in "bearing down" may risk rupture of membranes or stimulate premature labor.

If you are a single mother or your partner is unable to attend childbirth classes with you, you may want to practice relaxation and breathing exercises at home using a tape recorder. Begin by reading the relaxation sequence on page 31. Your voice on tape will condition you to respond to yourself as coach. When talking into the tape recorder, give yourself directions; then pause to follow them, similar to practicing in class.

Breathing exercises can also be practiced in this manner while you are sitting up, lying on your side, semi-reclining, or walking around. Begin by using Slow Chest Breathing. The tape should tell you, "Contraction begin. Take a deep cleansing breath, relax when you exhale, use a focal point. 5 seconds . . . 10 seconds . . . 15 seconds (and so on) until contraction ends. Take a cleansing breath and relax." Repeat this sequence 5 times, giving yourself a minute or two between contractions.

Use the same pattern for Accelerated Chest Breathing, Pant-Blow Breathing and pushing. Record five 70–90 second contractions using each breathing exercise. Give yourself praise and encouragement. Remind yourself to deal with one contraction at a time and to change positions frequently.

POSITIONS OF COMFORT DURING LABOR

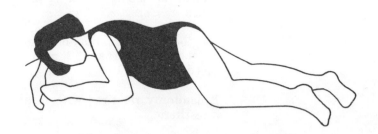

SIDE OR SIMS POSITION

Curl up on either side. Bend both knees making sure the upper knee is in front of the lower one. This puts the weight of the baby on the bed. Make sure all joints are flexed, not straight. This position is very good for total relaxation and allows the labor partner to apply pressure to the lower back if it is painful.

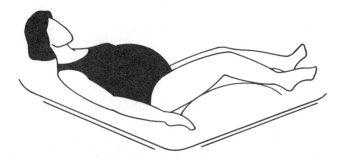

RECLINING CHAIR POSITION

Have the head and lower parts of the bed elevated to a half sitting position. Let your arms and legs fall apart on the bed. Effleurage (gently rhythmic rubbing of the abdomen) can best be done in this position.

TAILOR SITTING

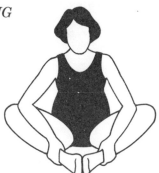

This is an excellent alternate position during active labor. Lean slightly forward to take the weight of baby off the spine. (See page 7)

RELAXATION TECHNIQUES AND EXERCISES

These techniques are extremely important to condition your body in the art of relaxation. Labor is strenuous. The uterus will be working very hard during labor. Your task will be to allow it to work freely while you keep the rest of your body deliberately relaxed. These exercises will help you develop muscle control and enable you to relax your entire body when commanded to do so.

Your labor partner should practice these exercises with you. It is impossible for you to check on your own relaxation since you will be involved in your labor. However, your partner will see these tensions immediately and can help you relax and conserve your energy.

This endeavor will require considerable discipline and teamwork from both of you. Therefore the labor partner must be as committed to the effort as you are. Lie in a comfortable position, on the floor or in the bed.

Follow a sequence of tensing one new body part each time. Start with your toes and progress in the following order:

Toes—lower legs—upper legs—buttocks—abdomen—shoulders—arms—fingers—face. For example:

1. Tense your toes. Hold them. Relax your toes.
2. Tense your toes, tense your lower legs. Hold them. Relax your lower legs, relax your toes.
3. Tense your toes, tense your lower legs, tense your upper legs. Hold them. Relax your upper legs, relax your lower legs, relax your toes.
4. Tense your toes, tense your lower legs, tense your upper legs, tense your buttocks. Hold them. Relax your buttocks, relax your upper legs, relax your lower legs, relax your toes.
5. . . . and so on to include the above mentioned body parts.
6. Take a deep breath releasing it completely through the mouth. This is referred to as a "cleansing breath."

The above relaxation exercise is called progressive relaxation and is most effective in achieving complete relaxation.

Learn how to tense a single body part, such as an arm, fist, leg or toes while keeping the rest of the body relaxed. For example:

1. Tense your right arm. Hold it a few seconds.
2. Relax your right arm.
3. Tense your left leg. Hold it.

4. Relax your left leg.
5. . . . etc. to include all body parts.
6. Take a deep cleansing breath and relax.

You will soon realize how difficult it is to work with one part of your body while keeping the rest of your body relaxed. It will demand your utmost and absolute concentration. By practicing these exercises at least once a day, you will become more aware of your body, establish a source of teamwork with your partner and learn to conserve your energy for your labor.

A relaxation technique being used with increasing frequency is called touch relaxation. In this form of relaxation, the labor partner will gently stroke the tense body part; and the mother will gradually relax this area. This stroking motion relieves the tension. By saying the word "relax" while stroking, the partner gives a verbal as well as a tactile (touch) cue.

In labor, the skills you both have acquired during weeks of practice will help you relax the tension by using gentle stroking. This is especially important when trying to cope with the transition phase of labor or back labor.

BREATHING EXERCISES FOR LABOR AND BIRTH

The three basic breathing exercises are simple and easy to use under the stress and anxiety of labor. There are four important points to remember:

1. Relaxation exercises help relax your body at a time when you may otherwise tense up and "fight" the contraction. Instead of gritting your teeth, digging your fingernails into the bed or curling your toes, you will be able to concentrate on your breathing exercise, automatically helping your body to relax.

2. Since you will work together as a team, it is equally important for your labor partner to be completely familiar with the breathing patterns so he or she can coach you during labor.

3. Breathing exercises will not eliminate all the discomfort of childbirth. They will condition you to react to the discomfort by concentrating on breathing. These exercises demand your utmost concentrated effort and activity.

4. You cannot fail or become a failure in these techniques. Your goal is to be able to contribute as much as you can in giving birth. There is no absolute measure that you must reach. Just do the best you can! Work to cope with each contraction to the best of your ability under the circumstances.

BREATHING EXERCISE NO. 1—Slow Chest Breathing

Slow, deep chest breathing is most useful during the early phase of the first stage of labor. Begin breathing exercises when you absolutely have to for maintaining relaxation. Doing breathing exercises too early wastes valuable energy. At the beginning and end of each breathing pattern, take a deep breath in and exhale completely. This cleansing breath is important to the body's oxygen and carbon dioxide balance.

Take a slow, deep breath in through the nose, then exhale slowly through pursed lips. If you are doing this exercise correctly, your chest should gently rise and fall.

You must find your own rate of speed. Remember that the faster you breathe the more exhausted you become. Also, try to take in and let out equal amounts of air to maintain the balance of oxygen in your body.

Example:

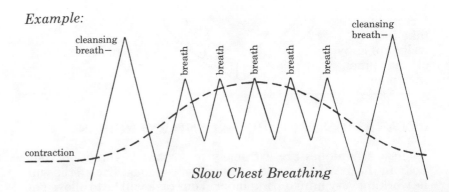

Slow Chest Breathing

BREATHING EXERCISE NO. 2—*Accelerated Chest Breathing*

When the contractions become more intense and it becomes difficult to maintain control of them, a more rapid shallow chest breathing may be used.

Take a cleansing breath. Then begin short, shallow "ha" or "he" breaths at a comfortable rate of speed. As the contraction subsides, slow down your rate of breathing to avoid hyperventilating. Symptoms of hyperventilation are numbness and tingling around the mouth, fingers and toes, dizziness and nausea. To correct the imbalance of oxygen and carbon dioxide which is the cause of these symptoms, simply rebreathe your own air by cupping your hands over your mouth or breathing into a paper bag.

Try to balance your breathing by taking equal amounts of air in and out. Use your chest muscles. You may want to place your hand on your chest to feel the movement.

Accelerated chest breathing is more difficult than slow chest breathing since it is more rapid and shallow. You may need to change the rate of your breathing several times within one contraction to adapt to the increasing and decreasing intensity.

Practice regularly to find out what rate is comfortable for you. This type of breathing is usually easier to do in labor during an actual contraction.

This second breathing exercise is sometimes eliminated and only exercises one and three are used. Some programs place less emphasis on breathing techniques or simplify the breathing patterns. Using only two breathing patterns may help the laboring mother, her partner and the nursing staff master the techniques and utilize them under the stress of labor. Accelerated chest breathing is most helpful during the middle phase of labor between the time the cervix is 4 and 7 centimeters dilated. Once transition is reached, switch to pant-blow breathing.

BREATHING EXERCISE NO. 3—*Pant-Blow*

This pant-blow pattern of breathing is a more shallow rapid type of breathing and is used when the contractions become extremely long and difficult to manage. This will happen during the transition phase of labor when the cervix is almost fully dilated. Although this phase usually lasts only a short time, it is quite intense and exhausting.

Take a slow deep cleansing breath. Then take three light shallow breaths, almost like the panting of a dog. Count the breaths 1, 2, 3 and then take a 4th shallow breath, and, as you exhale, blow out through your mouth as though you were blowing out a candle. Immediately take another four shallow breaths and blow out the fourth forcefully.

Example:

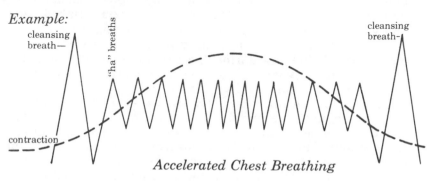

Accelerated Chest Breathing

Rate increases as contraction reaches a peak
then decreases as contraction subsides.

Example:

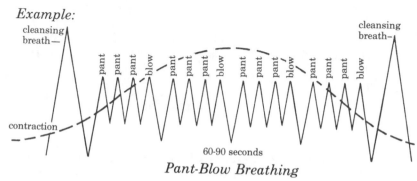

Pant-Blow Breathing

Keep up this pattern—pant pant pant blow, pant pant pant blow, as long as the contraction lasts and finish with a deep cleansing breath.

BREATHING EXERCISE FOR PUSHING

After the cervix is completely dilated and effaced, the baby is ready to pass down through the birth canal. The hardest work of labor is over and you can now push. The birth of the baby is very near, and you can now be active!

To push most effectively, while the contraction is building up, take two deep cleansing breaths; then take a third deep breath in through your mouth and hold it, pushing toward the vagina. Hold your breath for as long as you are comfortable; exhale, inhale again and hold it. Push only during the contraction. Between contractions, lie down and relax completely.

Please do not practice vigorous pushing during pregnancy—just practice holding your breath and very gently, bear down.

Example:

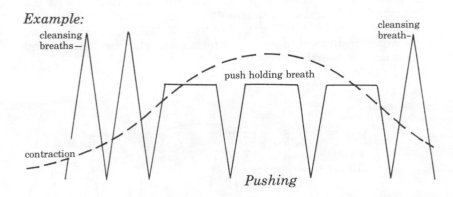

There are several positions in which you may push. You may try both positions until you find the one most comfortable and effective for you.

1. *Semi-sitting:* Prop your shoulders up to a 35-40 degree angle with pillows or support from labor partner. Draw legs up to about a 90 degree angle. Hold knees apart with your hands.

Hold your breath. Exert pressure by using your diaphragm and abdominal muscles in a forward and downward direction. If you pull your legs up too high, the natural curve of the pelvis will point toward the ceiling rather than gently outward. There may also be unnecessary tautness of the perineum, which may increase the need for episiotomy.

2. *Side-lying:* Draw your upper leg to hip level. Hold your knee or prop your foot on bed rail. As the contraction builds, round shoulders, lower head and push. This position is especially effective for back labor. Some women also find it easier to push in this position.

Your first pushes will bring your baby down the birth canal so that a small area of scalp or hair will be visible at the opening. Your baby's head will recede back between contractions. As you continue pushing, the head will almost be ready to come out or will "crown." At this time the doctor will want to guide the head out between contractions and may ask you not to bear down. This may be very difficult to do unless you begin panting or blowing. Open your mouth and begin breathing shallow short breaths or blow out as though you were blowing out candles. You may also be asked to just pant or blow if the cervix is not quite fully dilated and you are finding it difficult to refrain from pushing.

Some authorities are questioning the safety of vigorous prolonged breath holding during the second stage of labor. It is thought that too vigorous pushing may cause increased intercranial pressure and fetal hypoxia.

If more gentle pushing is advocated by your doctor, midwife, or labor nurse, try exhaling slowly by making an "s" or an "m" sound as you bear down during a contraction. Your diaphragm and abdominal muscles will bear down on the uterus, causing the baby to descend through the cervix and birth canal. You may also be instructed to release a small amount of air before holding your breath to push with a contraction.

Regardless of the method you are instructed to use, the important things to remember are:
—Relax your pelvic floor as in Kegel exercises.
—Relax your legs and buttocks.
—Keep your shoulders elevated; strong arms or pillows work fine.
—The urge to push will become strongest when the pressure from the baby's head increases.

PRACTICE THESE BREATHING EXERCISES EACH DAY. Rehearse in your mind the labor and birth of your baby. Start with the first stage, effacement and dilation and continue through transition, pushing and birth. Condition yourself to know your role so completely that you will perform controlled breathing and relaxation automatically and effortlessly.

Prepare yourself for various types of labors. Your labor may be one that progresses very rapidly from one phase or stage to another. If this is the case, use whatever breathing exercise is easiest and provides the greatest comfort. It is quite possible that slow chest breathing may be all that is necessary to carry you right through to transition or pant blow type breathing.

It is common for a woman to have dilated quite far, up to 5 or 6 centimeters over several days, with very little discomfort except for some backache or menstrual-like cramps. In this case, you may find your active labor to be intense from the very start; and you may need to go into rapid chest breathing or pant-blow immediately.

SPECIAL MESSAGE FOR THE LABOR PARTNER!

Whether you are the baby's father or another loving and caring labor partner, you are very important! Your presence eliminates a common fear of the laboring woman—the fear of being left alone.

The presence of a loving, caring and supporting person with a mother during labor makes a profound impact on the length of her labor, the amount of pain she experiences and the state of her emotions. Ideally, this person is the baby's father, who has also been the primary source of support throughout the pregnancy. However, should the baby's father not be present, the expectant mother will be strengthened by the presence of a friend, her mother or another relative.

It is not accidental that those sharing in the childbirth experience develop such an attachment and tenderness for the newborn infant, that each one feels an investment in the infant's future. This responsibility is shared by whoever is privileged to take part—nurses, physicians or other persons witnessing the birth and, of course, the mother and her partner.

Because your presence with your partner in labor is such an important and supportive role, you should be familiar with the processes of labor. The information in the following guide is divided into five major sections: Early Labor, Active Labor, Transition, Second Stage and After the Birth. You will find it arranged in the same manner as the labor guide.

You may want to take these guides with you to the hospital; there may be time to read them over if the labor is a slow one.

EARLY LABOR

1. Be calm and have confidence in yourself. Remember your presence and companionship is your most important contribution.

2. If her contractions begin at night, urge her to sleep as much as possible. If they begin during the daytime, help her to pass the time by relaxing, talking, reading, playing cards, watching television, walking, etc. The exception would be if the membranes rupture. Even if there are no other signs of labor, call your doctor immediately.

3. Do not force her to go to bed. Most women prefer to sit in a comfortable chair with head, arms and legs supported or walk about for brief periods, pausing momentarily to support the body and relax with contractions.

4. Your partner should not start her controlled breathing until she feels the need. When she does, her breathing should be deep, slow and even. At this stage of her labor she will probably be in control of herself and her breathing, and a few words of praise from you is all that is needed at this time.

5. Know in advance the route to the hospital. Approximate how long it will take, note the parking facilities and decide what entrance to use day or night. When you start, drive carefully and avoid sudden stops and rapid turns. There's plenty of time. Remind her to relax and breathe slowly and evenly with the contractions.

6. Tell the nurse you have been to class and you plan to stay with your partner (if this is the case). In some hospitals, be prepared to stay in the father's waiting room while she is being admitted. You will be allowed to join her later.

ACTIVE LABOR

1. Contractions are definitely closer, stronger and more determined. Your partner no longer wants to chat and becomes quiet and more preoccupied with her labor. Do not disturb or distract her during a contraction for they demand her deepest concentration.

2. A quiet, subdued environment will aid her ability to relax. Avoid bright lights shining in her eyes, excessive chatter and movements in the room.

3. The position of your partner is important to her physical comfort and ability to relax. In the back relaxation position, the head of the bed should be elevated about 45 degrees, and knees should be flexed slightly (contour-chair position). In the side relaxation position, the bed should be flat with your partner on her side, top leg forward, bent slightly and supported with a pillow. Help her change positions when she tires of one, elevate or lower the bed and rearrange the pillows.

4. WOMEN IN LABOR APPRECIATE LITTLE GESTURES OF COMFORT. A cool washcloth to wipe her face and neck, a wet washcloth to moisten her dry lips, a soothing backrub, a few ice chips, if permitted are all appreciated.

5. OFFER FREQUENT WORDS OF ENCOURAGEMENT. Such words as, "You're doing nicely," "Wonderful," "Keep up the good work," do not come often enough. The use of positive suggestions such as "Your contraction is at its peak and will soon be letting up" may help.

6. HELP HER WITH HER CONTROLLED BREATHING. Remember this is her best tool to aid her relaxation and enables her to work with the uterine contractions. Remind her to keep breathing as deeply and as slowly as possible and to keep her mind on her breathing. She should use the complete slow and deep breathing as long as possible, changing to rapid chest breathing and then pant-blow breathing when necessary.

TRANSITION

This period of her labor (8-10 cm.) is the most demanding. The contractions are long, strong and one after another. She may be irritable, discouraged and temporarily panic. She will need your help now more than ever and will need someone to give her directions as to what to do with each contraction.

1. Remind her this period is short. Relief will come with the second stage. Encourage her to think only of one contraction at a time and that there is a rest period after each contraction.

2. If she has had medication, she may doze between contractions and be confused when she awakens. Speak to her when the contraction starts and tell her to keep her eyes open and her attention on whoever is guiding her.

3. If she panics and momentarily loses control, speak to her in a firmer voice saying, "Breathe with me—pant pant pant blow, pant pant pant blow, keep it up, keep it even, just a little bit longer," etc. until the contraction is over.

4. If she has increasing low backache during the contraction, the firm steady pressure of the palm of your hand will ease the discomfort.

5. A catch in her breathing or a sensation that she cannot breathe with the urge to move her bowels signals the onset of the second stage of labor (expulsion stage). Urge her to continue panting until the urge is strong and irresistible. Make sure the nurse and doctor know she feels like pushing.

SECOND STAGE

The expulsion or pushing stage will bring mixed feelings of surprise, relief and joy. Surprised by the strange and indescribable power and joy signals anticipation of birth and a feeling that she can now actively participate in bringing the birth about. She needs to be reassured that these sensations are normal and that pushing will bring relief. She will also need DIRECT GUIDANCE as to what to do.

1. When the doctor or nurse gives her the 'go-ahead' to push, encourage her to take two deep breaths, hold the third (lips closed), lift her head (places diaphragm down on uterus) and bear down firmly and steadily. When needed, she can let out and take in another breath and continue pushing throughout the contraction. Counting out loud with each pushing breath is helpful.

2. Informing her of her progress encourages her to keep pushing during each contraction.

3. When the nurse signals it is time to prepare for the birth of the baby, **remain calm**. You may then put on the special attire needed to cover your clothing so the birth environment will be kept as clean as possible. This may include putting on a "scrub suit" or coveralls, cap, mask and shoe covers.

4. In the delivery or birthing room you will want to stay near your partner's side. Keep her informed of what is happening and repeat the doctor's instructions to her. Your voice is familiar and she will respond to it readily. Do not be alarmed at the "hustle and bustle" of nurses preparing for the birth and care of the infant. You may stand to watch the birth if you wish, or perhaps there will be a mirror to help both of you see your baby's birth. Try to eat a sandwich or snack while you are working with your partner

during labor. Full stomachs are much less likely to feel nauseated.

5. Birth is a moment of great emotion, and a father who has seen the birth of his own child is usually exhilarated and excited. Most partners describe the experience as "fantastic." "I could hardly believe I was seeing my own child come into the world." A father's presence is important not only for the father himself but for the mother, who needs him to be available, both physically and psychologically.

6. After birth, your partner may be kept in the delivery, or birthing room or a recovery room for a period for observation of her blood pressure, bleeding, etc. Many hospitals provide time for the new family to be together immediately following birth.

AFTER THE BIRTH

1. Immediately after birth it is very important that the two of you have close contact with your new baby. These first few days of contact are the beginning of an important emotional bond not only between you and your baby but between the two of you. Scientific evidence strongly suggests that during the immediate post partum period, new mothers in particular are highly sensitive to contact with their newborns.

2. Feel free to hold, touch and fondle your baby. Mother may be more comfortable curling up on her side where she can look at baby's face and snuggle close to him. Lying skin-to-skin under a warm blanket is a wonderful way to keep both mother and baby warm and satisfy their need to remain together following birth.

3. A picture may be taken of the new family to capture the moment forever. Other children at home can enjoy the birth also when given a picture of the event.

4. If the baby is premature or ill at birth and is being cared for in an Intensive Care Nursery, you are encouraged to visit the baby as soon as possible. You will want to touch and hold your baby if conditions permit.

5. Many hospitals offer "rooming-in" with the baby in the mother's room for some or all of the time. This closeness helps both mother and father become familiar with their new son or daughter and learn caretaking tasks gradually.

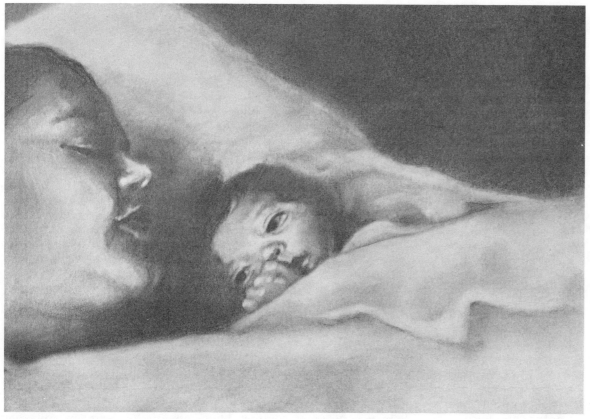

CESAREAN CHILDBIRTH

Cesarean birth is a term whose time has come. Many parents and health professionals are recognizing the fact that *a baby is born* by cesarean birth rather than *a mother has had a cesarean section*. Cesarean birth is no longer thought of as only a surgical procedure.

No doubt about it the cesarean birth rate has tripled in the last decade to a rate of 18 percent of all births. In fact, approximately a half million women in the United States now deliver their babies by Cesarean. These statistics encourage all expectant parents to learn about current and future trends surrounding Cesarean birth.

Why are so many babies born by cesarean? The reason may lie with the mother or the baby or sometimes both. If, for example, a mother's pelvic bones are too small or the baby too large to fit through a normal size pelvis, it would be best for both mother and baby if the birth would take place through the abdomen. Some obstetricians now consider cesarean to be safest for babies in a breech position, especially first babies. Frequently diagnostic tests are done to determine the exact size of the pelvis and the baby and to measure the effects of uterine contractions on the baby's heart rate. Rarely can a pelvic exam done early in pregnancy definitely determine whether you will have a cesarean birth or not.

Other reasons making a cesarean more safe for either mother or baby are toxemia of pregnancy, diabetes or accidents of the placenta. For example in placenta previa, the placenta partially or totally covers the cervix; or in placenta abruptio, the placenta separates partially or totally from the wall of the uterus. Fetal distress, often detected by monitoring the baby's heart rate, and failure of labor to progress are reasons for a cesarean birth sometimes after labor has already begun. And finally, "repeat" cesarean births, when the risk of rupture of the uterus is too great to permit natural labor, account for a substantial portion of cesarean births.

A number of obstetricians and parents are concerned about the growing rate of cesarean birth and have recommended guidelines be set up that will lower the rate of Cesareans. For example, in some areas, women with previous cesarean births are given the option of a vaginal delivery if their previous uterine incision was the low horizontal type which rarely ruptures and heals easily.

Also, some of the increase in Cesarean birth has been for women whose labor does not progress normally. Sometimes slow labor can be improved by encouraging a woman to walk during her labor or to sleep for several hours to give her body a rest. These measures should be tried before resorting to a Cesarean unless of course the baby is in trouble.

When a repeat Cesarean is deemed safest for you in your situation, it is usually scheduled near your due date. If your due date is questionable, several tests may be performed to more accurately determine it. Two of the most common tests are ultrasound and 24 hour urine estriol level. (See pg 46) As in the case of any diagnostic procedure, ask your physician to explain the nature and purpose of the test as well as the benefits, risks, and costs.

What can you expect if you give birth by cesarean? Many parents are unnecessarily frightened because they haven't allowed themselves to think of it as an alternative to a vaginal birth. Cesarean birth is not abnormal, and in most cases, the mother and baby will be in better health because of it. Sound medical practice dictates that a cesarean birth *never* be done solely for the convenience of the physician or mother. (The decision in favor of a cesarean birth is best arrived by mutual agreement between parents and the physician, and with as much discussion as possible.)

Physical preparations are made similar to those for a vaginal birth. Your abdomen and pelvic area will be shaved and a small tube called a catheter will be passed into your bladder to keep it empty. You will have a more thorough physical exam and an anesthesiologist will discuss with you the types of anesthetics available. Together you can decide which one—general, spinal or epidural—will be best for you and your baby. Most likely an intravenous fluid feeding will be started either by the anesthesiologist or nurse.

The cesarean may be done in the delivery room or operating room. After you are positioned, washed and draped, the baby will be delivered through incisions in your abdomen and uterus. Surprisingly, your baby will be born in about five to ten minutes. You will be awake with a spinal or epidural anesthesia and will hear the baby cry, see him, and touch him soon after birth. When general anesthesia has been administered, the reunion of mother and baby can take place as soon as the mother is conscious, perhaps shortly after returning to her room from the recovery area. Several hours will have elapsed between the time you first entered the operating or delivery room until you are back in your hospital room.

Extra time and care in the hospital are needed after a cesarean childbirth. You can expect a five to seven day hospital stay, some incisional discomfort, and some degree of abdominal gas. Walking and taking extra fluids and pain medications as needed will help you be more comfortable. Your stitches will probably be removed before you go home but can be removed later in your physician's office.

More specific details about preparation for a cesarean birth and the procedure itself are often part of your childbirth program. Films or slides showing cesarean births can help prepare parents for a possible or scheduled cesarean. You may want to talk to parents who have had a cesarean birth to learn first hand about this type of childbirth.

Should your baby be born by cesarean, ask about the possibility of your partner remaining with you during the birth or being together in the recovery room afterwards. The family is bonded closer together when parents can see and hold the baby as soon after the birth as possible. After all, a cesarean is a birth.

GUIDE TO MEDICATIONS & ANESTHETICS USED DURING CHILDBIRTH

There are almost as many variations in the types of medications and anesthetics that may be used during labor and birth as there are types of childbirth itself. Each woman is unique and has different needs. Some will desire or need no drugs; others will need only a few, and still others will demand they be given.

It is the philosophy of many hospitals that each mother be cared for according to her own individual needs and requests, with the understanding that she be educated and informed of the risks and benefits with the use of medications during childbirth. During your prenatal visits, discuss with your physician or midwife the types of medications they generally use. Let them know what your preferences are. You may well favor the use of no medications or one particular type, but it's best to be flexible, knowing that not all medications are right for all situations.

Above all, remember that it is not necessary for you to achieve perfection or prove your competency during childbirth. You do not "pass or fail"; however, you do participate and give birth, regardless of the style of childbirth or use of medication.

Although there are additional drugs that could be added to this guide, their use is so infrequent that only the most widely used drugs are included. Your physician or nurse can further clarify the types of medications used most frequently in your hospital and geographic area. You may use this book as a reference and circle or underline specific information if it is yours to keep.

TYPE	NAME	PURPOSE/BENEFITS	POSSIBLE DISADVANTAGES
Narcotics	Demerol Nisentil Morphine Mepergan Talwin	Usually given in middle of first stage of labor (once labor pattern regular and strong). Demerol has longer lasting effect; Nisentil acts more rapidly but has short duration. May be given in the muscle or I.V. Takes edge off discomfort; enhances relaxation. May cause sleep between contractions.	May slow or stop labor if given too early. If given too late, may cause respiratory distress in newborn. May cause nausea or drop in mother's blood pressure.
Tranquilizer	Atarax Vistaril Largon Sparine Phenergan Thorazine Compazine Valium Librium Equanil Miltown	Given in early to middle of first stage of labor if mother is tense, anxious, or agitated. May be given in conjunction with a narcotic to both relax and relieve pain. Given in muscle or I.V. Helps relaxation process; helps prevent mother from becoming extremely tense with contractions.	May cause dizziness, drowsiness, or drop in mother's blood pressure. Some cause loss of beat to beat variation in fetal heart tones, poor muscle tone, and hypothermia.

TYPE	NAME	PURPOSE/BENEFITS	POSSIBLE DISADVANTAGES
Barbiturate	Nembutal Seconal Chloral Hydrate Amytal Butisol Luminal	Usually given late evening or at night if mother is in very early labor or has ruptured membranes but no labor. Helps mother sleep a few hours prior to labor or induction of labor. Given orally in capsule or pill, I.M. or I.V.	Accentuates action of narcotics if given concurrently. Mother may feel groggy for several hours after taking a barbiturate. Infants born within several hours have significant amounts of drug in their body.
Anti-Secretory	Atropine Scopolomine	Helps to dry air passages for general anesthesia, especially for cesarean birth. Scopolomine produces "amnesia" and is not commonly used for obstetric purposes. Given in muscle or I.V.	Dry mouth, lips may dry and crack. When Scopolomine is combined with a narcotic, it produces a "twilight sleep." Both depress the central nervous system.
Regional Anesthesia using "caine" drugs such as Carbocaine Novacaine Pontocaine Blockain	Paracervical Block	A local anesthetic is injected into tissue on either side of cervix (at approximately 4 and 8 o'clock) to anesthetize the cervical area. Given when cervix is 3 cm dilated or more. Lasts ½ to 2 hours. Provides total or partial relief of deep pelvic discomfort due to dilatation of cervix.	Allergy to caine drugs prohibits its use. May not relieve back labor. May cause temporary slowing of baby's heart rate. If given too early, slows labor.
Metycaine Nesacaine Marcaine Nupercaine	Local	A local anesthetic is injected into perineal area to numb skin and underlying tissue before episiotomy is done.	May sting slightly when administered. Little or no adverse effect on mother or baby.
Citanest Xylocaine Procaine	Pudendal Block	Approximately ½ oz. of local anesthetic is injected deep into lower sides of vagina to numb perineum and labia; more extensive numbing than local. Relaxes perineum. Given only after complete dilatation or birth for repair.	Little or no adverse effect on mother or baby.

TYPE	NAME	PURPOSE/BENEFITS	POSSIBLE DISADVANTAGES
Regional Anesthesia (Cont.)	Saddle Block	A type of "low spinal." A local anesthetic mixed with a Dextrose solution is injected into the spinal canal while mother is in a sitting position. Numbed from the pubic area to toes. Can be given during labor and lasts for childbirth. Usually administered by obstetrician.	Usually necessitates the use of forceps as mother loses pushing sensation. May cause a drop in mother's blood pressure, which may affect baby also. The use of I.V.'s and lying flat 6-8 hours following birth help prevent headaches which might occur after spinal.
	Spinal Block	A local anesthetic mixed with Dextrose solution is injected into the spinal canal while mother is in a side lying position. Numbs area from above navel to toes. Can be used for vaginal childbirth. Slightly larger dosage used for cesarean.	May cause a drop in mother's blood pressure. Same restriction as for saddle block.
	Epidural Caudal	A local anesthetic is injected into the epidural space near the spinal cord. A small catheter may be placed in the space and the anesthetic agent administered through the catheter either in one or repeated dosages.	Skilled personnel necessary to administer epidural anesthesia and monitor mother's blood pressure. Loss of bearing down reflex may necessitate use of forceps. It may also prolong labor if started too early.
Inhalation	Nitrous Oxide	A fast acting gas inhaled during contractions just prior to birth or during expulsion of placenta. Gives excellent analgesia. Should be given with at least 25% oxygen. Mother may feel floating sensation and doze for several seconds. Usually given just during expulsion of head and in conjunction with local. Can be rapidly administered for emergency situations or for applying forceps.	Mother may feel she was asleep a long time. May dream or hear distorted sounds. May be unsafe to use if mother's stomach contains food or liquid. Most common anesthetic agent used for obstetrics in this country. Safe for baby if dose kept low and administered with sufficient oxygen.

TYPE	NAME	PURPOSE/BENEFITS	POSSIBLE DISADVANTAGES
Inhalation (Cont.)	Penthrane	Sweet fruity smelling gas inhaled just prior to birth. Falls sound asleep as long as needed. May be given for forceps delivery when spinal is contraindicated.	Not to be used if mother's stomach is full, except in dire emergencies. No depression of newborn if given in light amounts. Prolonged anesthesia produces newborn depression and may depress respiration, liver, kidney, and G.I. tract in mother.
	Fluothane Ether Cyclopropane Trilene Chloroform	All provide analgesia and varying levels of consciousness. Not commonly used for obstetric purposes.	Blood concentrations necessary to produce anesthesia frequently cause respiratory distress and fetal narcosis. Vomiting and aspiration of vomitus a grave complication when used in delivery.
General	Pentothal	Given I.V. for cesarean birth. Produces very rapid sleep; mother is completely scrubbed and draped before drug is given. Baby is delivered within 4-7 minutes to minimize effect of drug on baby. May be agent of choice when emergency cesarean is necessary.	Because absorption in fetal circulation is very rapid, this drug is not advisable for vaginal deliveries. Must be administered by a skilled anesthetist.
Oxytocics	Pitocin Oxytocin Syntocinon	Stimulates uterine contractions to induce or hasten labor. Also used postpartum to help uterus contract and decrease bleeding. Usually given in I.V. solution regulated by infusion or IVAC pump which insures exact uniform dosage. Fetal monitor is usually applied when Pitocin is used in labor.	Mother and baby must be observed closely; physician must be in hospital. Care must be taken not to overstimulate uterus. Contractions usually stronger, more intense and progress rapidly; mother may need more coaching and support. May cause drop in mother's blood pressure and irregularities in heart rate. Is also associated with increased incidence of jaundice in the newborn.
	Buccal Pitocin	Small tablets are dissolved between lip and gums (lining of mouth) given at timed intervals to stimulate or induce labor. Dosage can be discontinued by removing tablets and rinsing mouth.	If mother wears dentures, they must be removed first. Makes mouth coated and pasty. Same precautions as I.V. Pitocin.

TYPE	NAME	PURPOSE/BENEFITS	POSSIBLE DISADVANTAGES
Oxytocics (Cont.)	Ergotrate Methergine	Usually given orally but may be administered I.V. or in the muscle. Used immediately post-partum to prevent or regulate bleeding.	May cause cramping of uterus. May elevate mother's blood pressure.
Intravenous Solutions	Glucose Saline	May be indicated to help raise mother's blood pressure and provide energy or fluid vehicle to administer a drug.	Increase in urine output making it necessary to urinate more frequently. May restrict movement of arms or hands.

REFERENCES:

1. Clark, A. L., Affonso, D. *Childbearing: A Nursing Perspective,* E. A. Davis Co., Philadelphia, 1976.
2. Clausen, J. P., et. al. *Maternity Nursing Today,* McGraw-Hill Inc., New York, 1977.
3. Ericson, Avis J., *Medications Used During Labor and Delivery-A Resource for Childbirth Educators,* International Childbirth Education Association: Milwaukee, 1978.
4. Hassid, Patricia, *Textbook for Childbirth Educators,* Harper & Row Publishers, Inc., Hagerstown, 1978.
5. Reeder, S. R. et al. *Maternity Nursing,* J. B. Lippincott, Co., Philadelphia, 1976.

COMMONLY USED DIAGNOSTIC TESTS

Sometimes it is necessary to evaluate the health of the unborn child or determine its exact stage of development. Diagnostic tests are being used with increasing frequency, not only for pregnancies with complications, but for normal pregnancies as well. Physicians are doing them simply to verify such things as the due date or fetal maturity. A number of diagnostic tests can monitor the well-being of the fetus and the efficiency of the placenta.

So that you may be included in properly planning your care, here is some basic information about these tests. The information includes the benefits, and the risks involved with each test as well. They are mentioned here so you can become familiar with the different tests that may or may not be needed during your pregnancy. Do not be frightened by the technical matter or terms involved. The purpose of this information is to *inform* you, not *frighten* you. Perhaps it will relieve any apprehensions you may have should your physician recommend that a certain test be done.

AMNIOCENTESIS

Amniocentesis is the withdrawal of a small amount of amniotic fluid through a needle which has been inserted through the abdomen and uterus into the amniotic sac. The position of the fetus is carefully determined ahead of time and the heart rate checked frequently to make sure the procedure is not harmful. However, there is a slight risk of the fetus being punctured or infected or a miscarriage as the result of this procedure.

Tests are run on the cells that grow from cultures of the amniotic fluid. These tests can be time consuming and expensive so there should be a good reason for the amniocentesis—for example, diagnosing a genetic disorder such as Down's Syndrome or Tay-Sacks disease. Since amniocentesis can be done early in the pregnancy, parents may choose to end the pregnancy. However, they can also be reassured when their baby is not the victim of a family or chromosomal disorder.

In the last few months of pregnancy, amniocentesis may be done to determine the maturity of the baby's lungs. If the lungs are found to be immature, there is a greater chance the baby will develop respiratory distress after birth.

ESTRIOL MEASUREMENT

Estriol is a substance found during pregnancy in a mother's blood or urine. It is the result of the placenta's ability to change steroid precursors produced by the baby's adrenal glands into an estrogen product—hence the name estriol.

As pregnancy advances, the level of estriol in the mother's urine and blood increases; although amounts vary from day to day. Because of this variation, single measurements are of little value.

The urine estriol level is best determined by measuring the amount found in the urine in a 24 hour urine specimen. Frequently, a mother is asked to collect all urine for a 24 hour day, skip a day, then collect another 24 hour specimen. The urinary estriol test is less reliable if there is any problem with the mother's kidneys or liver.

Sometimes a blood estriol test is done together with or instead of a urine estriol test. This test would only indicate the immediate level rather than the efficiency of the placenta/fetus mechanism during the previous 24 hours.

It's important that the mother not be taking medication such as Ampicillin, Steroids or certain stool softeners since these drugs can interfere with accurate estriol levels. There are no hazards to the mother or baby in estriol testing.

Complications such as toxemia, intrauterine growth retardation and post maturity of the fetus are detectible through estriol testing. The major value of this test is to show whether the baby is in immediate danger or whether it may safely remain in the uterus for a while longer. This is very important when there is increasing risk to either mother or baby, and the physician must decide when to intervene.

ULTRASOUND

Ultrasound is a technique by which low intensity sound waves are sent through the mother's body and reflected back at tissue interfaces. These waves are then received by a transducer and translated onto an oscilloscope as a "picture" made of electrical blips.

A mother is asked to arrive for testing with a full bladder so that the uterus is pushed upward and is more visible. She will lie on her back, and mineral oil will be applied to her abdomen to help increase the conductivity. The ultrasound transducer is then passed over her abdomen, and the picture is formed on a small T.V.-like screen. The test usually takes between 15 and 60 minutes, depending on the position and activity of the fetus.

Ultrasound can reveal important information about the age and size of the fetus, where the placenta is located (important to know prior to amniocentesis and if abnormalities of the placenta are suspected), multiple pregnancies and some severe abnormalities. The size of the baby's head can be measured over a period of time to measure intrauterine growth and determine fetal size.

At the present time, no harmful effects from ultrasound have been reported. However, research is continuing in this area.

OXYTOCIN CHALLENGE TEST (O.C.T.)

If it is suspected that the placenta may not be functioning adequately, an O.C.T. or stress test may be done late in pregnancy and repeated on a weekly basis (or more often if necessary) until delivery. It stands to reason that a placenta that is not functioning properly before labor begins will further compromise the exchange of gases—mainly oxygen—after labor begins.

This test is done in the hospital where both mother and baby can be observed closely. A microphone which records the baby's heart beat and a small pressure gauge called a transducer are placed on the abdomen with an elastic belt. These devices are connected to the fetal monitor and provide a continuous recording of the baby's heart rate and uterine contractions.

After the monitor has been recording for about 15-30 minutes, an intravenous of sterile fluid will be started in the arm or hand. Then a drug called Pitocin is given very slowly in exact amounts to stimulate the uterus to contract. Some women do not feel the contractions, and others experience a cramping sensation in the lower abdomen or low backache.

The aim of the test is to stimulate three contractions within a ten minute period and to see how the baby and placenta react to the contraction. After an adequate reading has been obtained, the Pitocin is discontinued and the remaining intravenous fluid is given to dilute the drug remaining in the blood stream. The contractions gradually slow up and stop.

External monitoring is used with the O.C.T. since it doesn't require rupturing the membranes and invading the uterus.

If the fetal monitor shows that the baby's heart rate drops significantly after most contractions, this is an indication that the baby is endangered. Tests for fetal maturity such as the 24 hour urine estriol, which was previously mentioned, are then carried out to determine how soon the baby may be safely delivered. The stress test can also be repeated to rule out a false positive test result.

A negative O.C.T., where the heart rate does not show a uniform drop (see Fetal Monitoring) after contractions, means the fetus will safely remain in the uterus for at least one more week. Sometimes the efficiency of the placenta is doubtful (such as a mother with toxemia or diabetes) in which case O.C.T. should be repeated weekly until the end of pregnancy.

Since the test involves stimulating the uterus to contract, there is a slight risk of starting labor. Therefore, O.C.T. is not advisable for mothers who have a low-lying placenta (placenta previa) or when the risk of premature labor would be hazardous to the baby. If a mother has had a previous classical cesarean section (indicated by a scar on the uterus being vertical rather than horizontal), she would also be at risk if labor would begin.

Other complications, although rare, are hypotension (low blood pressure) and hyperstimulation of the uterus (meaning the uterus contracts frequently and for an abnormally long period of time). If hypotension develops during an O.C.T., this condition can usually be treated successfully by turning the mother on her left side. This side-lying position relieves pressure on the vena cava, a large vein leading to the heart. Hyperstimulation of the uterus is treated by immediately stopping the administration of the drug, Pitocin.

NON-STRESS TEST

A commonly used test to measure the response of the baby's heart rate to his or her activity is a non-stress test. The baby's heart rate is traced on a fetal monitor over a period of time and measured during periods of rest activity and stimulation. A poor result is when the heart rate does not respond normally to activity.

FETAL MONITORING

Electronic fetal monitoring is becoming more prevalent for both normal as well as complicated labors. Some centers monitor all mothers in labor; many monitor only high-risk labors or follow the protocol set by the individual physician.

The normal heart rate for the unborn child is between 120 and 160 beats per minute. A fetal monitor measures this as well as the contractions of the uterus and traces the readings on a graph paper. The tracing not only shows when the fetal heart rate falls below 120 or climbs above 160, but also variations of acceleration or deceleration that occur in relationship to the contractions. This relationship is essential information in assessing problems.

There are two types of monitoring—external and internal. External monitoring can be used prior to labor or early in labor when the membranes are not ruptured and the cervix undilated. A device which detects the fetal heartbeat, called a transducer, is attached to the mother's abdomen by an elastic strap or held in place under a stockingette. Another elastic strap attaches a pressure sensitive transducer to the abdomen (or it is also held in place under the same stockingette that holds the first transducer) to measure the strength of the contraction. The sound waves and amount of pressure picked up by the transducers are recorded on a strip of graph paper similar to the strip tape used in electrocardiograms.

The advantage of the external monitor is that it does not involve any entry into the body and is not likely to cause infection or injury. However, external monitoring may result in inaccurate tracings if the mother moves or the baby descends down the birth canal, making frequent adjustments necessary. Another disadvantage to external monitoring is that the best position for accurate tracings is for the mother to lie on her back, which may cause her blood pressure to drop and a late deceleration of the fetal heart rate.

Internal monitoring can be done after the cervix is dilated at least 2 centimeters and the membranes have ruptured. The fetal heart rate is measured by attaching a small spiral electrode directly to the baby's scalp. The contractions can be measured by placing a Teflon, fluid-filled catheter in the uterus to measure the pressure of the contraction. In some centers, the external pressure gauge is used in conjunction with the fetal scalp electrode, instead of placing a catheter inside the uterus.

The advantages of internal monitoring are several, the main one being increased accuracy. It also allows more freedom of movement for the mother and less chance of "supine hypotension," the lowering of the mother's blood pressure as the result of lying on her back.

However, certain disadvantages must be considered, such as the need to artificially rupture the membranes in order to apply the electrode. Rare complications such as fetal scalp infections and perforation of the uterus have been reported.

Fetal monitoring has undoubtedly rescued many infants who have suffered from lack of oxygen due to insufficient circulation in the placenta or compression of the umbilical cord. However, to date studies have failed to prove definitely that fetal outcome is improved with the routine monitoring of every labor.

Monitoring can be an extremely helpful tool for the labor partner, since the monitor can begin to register the contraction before the mother is aware of it. If her contractions are irregular or if she is sleeping between contractions, the labor partner can use the monitor to begin his or her coaching of a breathing technique. The labor partner can also tell the mother when the contraction has reached a peak and is diminishing. These kinds of verbal cues and encouragement are invaluable to both the mother who needs to know what is happening and the labor partner who needs to feel actively involved in the labor.

It helps to be able to see a fetal monitor and a sample tracing. At no time will you be expected to "read" the monitor or interpret a tracing; but if you would like more information about the variations in patterns and their significance, ask your childbirth educator, nurse or physician to review this with you. Talk to your physician about the current practices in your community or hospital and your feelings about monitoring during your labor.

EMERGENCY CHILDBIRTH

If labor progresses very rapidly or a mother fails to recognize that she is in the final stages of labor, a baby may be born at home or on the way to the hospital. Fortunately, in the vast majority of these childbirths, the labor is uncomplicated and the baby is healthy. Also, since no drugs or anesthetics have been given to the mother, the baby is more likely to be alert and to breathe immediately.

Nevertheless, many labor partners feel some uneasiness about being able to make it to the hospital in time. This section on emergency childbirth is written exclusively for you—the labor partner—since it is you who most likely will have to reassure the mother in an emergency childbirth.

A mother will almost always know if birth is imminent—take her word for it. She may feel the baby's head come down the birth canal, have a burning pressure or pain, and an uncontrollable urge to push.

If you are driving the car, resist the temptation to drive fast or take chances. The mother and baby are in far more danger from an accident than from childbirth. If it is safe to do so, pull off the road, put emergency flasher lights on and help the mother as she gives birth. In the event that a passing motorist stops to help, ask him to call an ambulance.

If you are at home, call an ambulance or have a neighbor do so. Regardless of where you are at the time of the emergency birth, try not to leave the mother alone unless you must go to get help.

Rely on your inner strength to remain as calm as possible. Calm the mother by using the slow chest or pant-blow breathing you learned in class. Then you are ready to assist in the following manner.

1. Have her lie down with newspapers, blanket or coat under her buttocks. Once the head is visible, have mother pant until head is born to prevent rapid expulsion or minimize tearing of tissue due to an excessively rapid birth.

2. Up until the time of delivery, your chief role is to make the mother as comfortable as possible, both physically and mentally. Reassure mother that she is doing a good job and you will get through the birth together.

3. If the baby's head is still covered by the membranes, looking as if it were in a cellophane bag, the membranes must be broken and removed from the baby's face. Use a car key or scissors to rupture them at the back of the baby's neck.

4. The baby's face, which will usually be looking toward the mother's rectum, can be wiped off with a clean cloth, and the mother should bear down strongly with the next contraction to deliver the baby's shoulders.

5. If the cord is around the baby's neck, the baby can usually be delivered through the loop and then the cord can be unwound. Sometimes it can be loosened and pulled over the baby's head before the body comes out of the birth canal.

6. Support the baby's head. Do not pull on baby; birth will be spontaneous.

7. When completely delivered, the baby should be held or placed on mother's abdomen with his face down or to the side to permit him to cough and drain out any mucus that may be in the nose or throat.

8. Almost all babies will breathe spontaneously after birth and are even more likely to be alert and active when the mother has not had drugs or anesthetics. Normally babies do not need to have their mouths wiped or cleaned out. However, if baby is white and limp, wipe out mouth with a clean cloth and vigorously rub his back or soles of his feet. Place him skin-to-skin with mother for warmth. Give artificial respiration if baby fails to breathe within 1½ minutes. However, use extreme care when administering mouth to mouth resuscitation to an infant.

Only the amount of air that can be held in your mouth when you blow out your cheeks should be blown into the baby's lungs. They are very small and are easily ruptured if too much air is administered.

9. Do not tie or cut the cord if you are on the way to the hospital or the doctor is coming soon.

10. Put the baby to the mother's breast if the cord is long enough. This will cause the uterus to contract and help expel the placenta.

11. Do not pull on the cord to loosen the placenta. The placenta may be delivered shortly after birth or not for 1 to 2 hours. If it does not deliver spontaneously wait for the doctor or proceed to the hospital, keeping baby, mother and placenta intact. If it is delivered, save placenta in a plastic bag or wrap it up in a towel or newspaper and take it along to the hospital for the doctor's inspection.

12. Rather free bleeding is to be expected at the time the placenta is delivered and immediately afterwards. This should not be more than about one cup. The suckling of the baby at the breast will minimize blood loss by stimulating the uterus to remain firm.

13. Keep mother and baby together and warm. If a doctor has been called, wait for his or her arrival. If you're in the car, go on to the hospital.

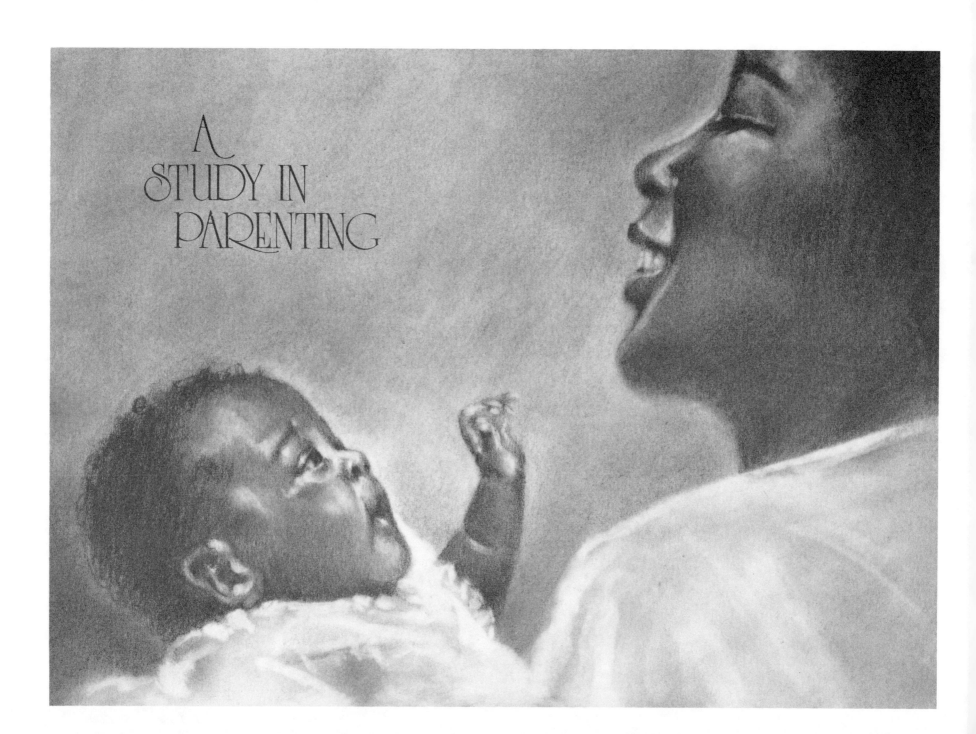

A
STUDY IN
PARENTING

Part III: A Study in Parenting

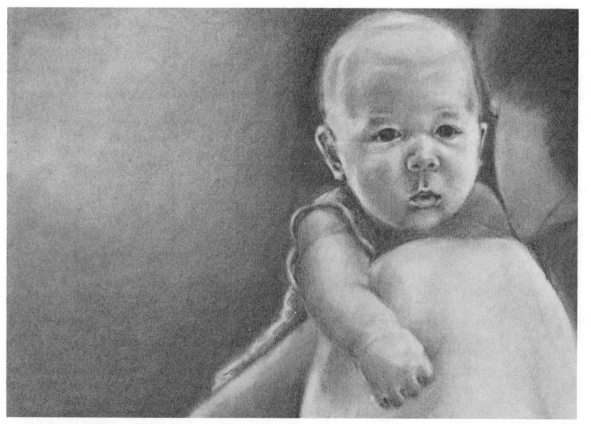

THE FIRST FEW MONTHS AT HOME

One of the most common responses to the question "After the birth I am most concerned about . . ." takes the form of another question—"What kind of parent will I be?" Those who already have children frequently ask, "Will I have the time to take care of another child?"

No doubt about it—parenting is hard work. Unlike labor and birth, which are over in a matter of hours, parenting is a lifetime experience. It's reassuring to know that it does get somewhat easier in time.

Those first few months of parenting seem to be the toughest ones. Major role changes and adjustments in lifestyle are inevitable. We seem to be less prepared to be a parent than for any other vocation.

Let's bring parenting into perspective by looking at those early months. If you can zero in on getting things ready ahead of time and anticipate ways of simplifying your lives, you will be able to relax and enjoy your baby to the fullest. Your baby will need your *full* time attention and care for a very short time in his lifetime, specifically, during the first few months.

In the following four sections of this manual you will find much information which may not be included in all prepared parenthood programs. Begin by reading all the sections, and then return to those areas that you would like to discuss either with your physician, nurse, childbirth educator or friends who have small children. You can expect some differences of opinion when discussing some areas, particularly in the section called "Family Contract." Just try to keep in mind that your style of parenting is uniquely yours. There are no perfect parents—just parents who keep trying to be good ones.

When you first get home from the hospital, you will probably need to spend the first week doing much the same as you did in the hospital—resting frequently, staying dressed in a comfortable robe and slippers and taking care of your own body needs. Warm water soaks or "sitz baths" once or twice a day can help comfort and heal the episiotomy. Heat from a lamp placed next to your bed can help dry and heal sore nipples and bottom, or try gently air drying those areas with a hair dryer set on a "warm" temperature.

The discharge from the healing uterus, called lochia, should be dark in color and will decrease in amount by the time your baby is four days old. If it increases in amount or suddenly becomes bright red again, it means you are exerting yourself too much and need to stay off your feet for a day or two. Call your physician if the increase or bright color continues for more than a day or two. It may mean that a piece of the placenta or membranes still remain in the uterus, and this will prevent it from healing properly. If this is the reason for your bleeding, you may have to be hospitalized for a D & C (dilatation and curretage).

Make an appointment with your physician for a postpartum checkup. Some physicians advise you to be examined four weeks after your baby is born, and some say five or six. Perhaps you will want to be examined prior to resuming sexual intercourse to make certain you have sufficiently healed with no signs of infection. You may want to discuss a method of birth control at this time, also.

HOUSEHOLD HELP

Whether this is your first or fourth child, you will need some type of household help for the first week or two at home. You will be able to care for yourself and the baby; but leave meals, dishes, ironing, cleaning and care of the older children to someone else. Generally speaking, a "baby nurse" is not necessary, especially if you are given the opportunity to care for your baby while you're in the hospital.

Husbands sometimes take vacation time and will provide the help that is needed. Many couples have said that with the first child they appreciated the opportunity to be alone during this time. Relatives (mothers, mothers-in-law or sisters) often enjoy helping. Just be sure you are comfortable with whoever is coming in to help. Remember, although their advice is "well-meaning," the final management of the baby is up to you.

Friends often ask how they can help and will appreciate direct suggestions. Caring for other children in the family, shopping, bringing in meals and ironing are all things which can be helpful to you.

High school or college students can supervise older children through the later afternoon, evening meal and preparation for bedtime.

Hired help is available through agencies, but they should be contacted early. Most agencies differentiate between a straight baby-sitting rate and a child and home care rate (rate according to ability to pay). The child and home care rate includes child care plus light housework, such as making beds, dusting, cooking, doing dishes and laundry. Most agencies will not do heavy house cleaning or provide transportation for the children. When contacting the agency, ask for references; and, if possible, have an interview with the person planning to come.

MEAL PLANNING

During the last few months of your pregnancy, you can save time and effort by planning or preparing meals ahead.

1. Write out one or two weeks of menus for simple, easily prepared meals by using frozen, canned or other convenience foods.

2. Bake double size casseroles and freeze one for later.

3. Make your own nutritious T.V. dinners and freeze them.

4. Check restaurants in your area that have carry-out dinners or that will deliver.

5. Consider using grocery, milk and bread delivery services temporarily.

6. Take your friends' offers to help seriously and ask them to bring in a meal.

7. If you're bottle feeding, consider using prepared formula for the first week or two.
8. Dishwashing can be kept at a minimum by using paper plates and paper cups.

Rest is essential for the new mother. Problems of adjustment to the baby are often aggravated when the mother is not getting sufficient rest.

Visitors can be tiring and the responsibility of restricting visitors often becomes the father's job. Try to restrict hospital visitors to the grandparents. The first day at home with a new baby can be confusing. Experienced parents have found a NO VISITOR policy, including grandparents, allows the new parents that important time of being alone and settling in with their baby. Visitors should be limited the first week at home to close friends you invite. Do not be afraid to admit fatigue, go to bed and rest. Staying in your night clothes the first week reminds people you need rest and they should know not to stay too long. It also helps to remind you that you should spend your time resting in bed and not working in the kitchen.

A rest period during the day is desirable for the next 3-6 months, especially to replace sleep lost at night. RESTING WHEN THE BABY NAPS is an excellent policy but one that is difficult for the new mother to learn. A relaxed and rested mother is more important to the smooth functioning of the household than clean floors or ironed clothes.

To avoid disturbances, take the phone off the hook; put a "sleeping note" on the door; and let friends know when you will be resting.

If you live in a two-story house, provide a resting area for yourself on the first floor and a dressing and sleeping area (car bed or carriage can be used) for the baby on both floors. To take advantage of the extra rest you need, lie down to feed the baby.

LAUNDRY

Using disposable diapers or diaper service for the first 4-6 weeks will save you time and energy. The cost of diaper service is usually less than using disposable diapers.

If you are using commercial laundromats, it is good policy to wash a load of your own clothes before the infant's as you do not know what was previously washed in the machine. Rinse baby clothes thoroughly, especially the diapers.

POSTPARTUM EXERCISES

One of the best things you can do for YOU is to set aside some time for yourself each day. You'll feel much more relaxed and less irritable if you pay attention to your own needs during this time when demands upon you are great.

Exercise is a good way to rebuild and tone your body as well as relieve some of the stress or tension you may experience as you adjust to your new lifestyle.

Start by resuming the Kegel exercise you practiced during pregnancy. Its real benefit will be felt now as you contract and pull up the vaginal muscles. Count to five as you tighten and pull inward; then, count again as you slowly release. Kegel exercises can be started immediately after childbirth and continued daily through life.

Abdominal contraction can also be started the day you give birth. Tighten abdominal muscles without holding your breath. Keep muscles tight for a few seconds, then relax. Your abdomen is likely to be loose and flabby at first—start gently, and gradually increase the vigor of the exercise each day.

After a week or so you may wish to add several more exercises. Use caution, however, if you are bleeding heavily or if you have been advised not to exercise for a medical reason.

Head raising: Lie on the floor or bed with your knees bent. Tense your abdominal muscles, and lift your head and shoulders. Hold for a count of 5; then, fall back and relax. Repeat 4 times the first week; then, gradually increase to 10 times.

Leg raising: Lie on the floor or bed with your left knee bent and right leg straight. Slowly lift your right leg as high as you can, keeping it straight; then slowly lower it to the bed. Next, do the same thing, lifting your left leg while your right knee is bent. Repeat 5 times the first week; then gradually increase to 10 times.

Touching knees: Also, while lying on the floor or bed, bend both knees and keep your feet flat. Slowly reach your hands upward and touch your knees for a few seconds; then slowly relax back to your resting position. Repeat 4 to 5 times the first week; then, gradually increase to 10 times.

After 4 to 6 weeks at home, you may want to begin a more vigorous exercise program. Taking your baby for walks, joining a swim program for tots, or exercising with your baby are excellent ways to keep your body fit and to enjoy your baby at the same time. You may also want to resume the body building exercises you used during pregnancy—see pages 7 and 8.

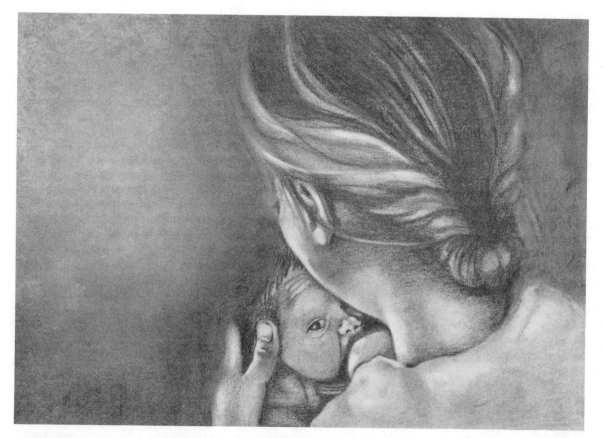

FEEDING YOUR BABY AN ACT OF LOVE

Babies need to feel loved and cared for. They learn to trust those around them if their needs are met rather promptly and consistently.

One of your baby's most pressing needs is for food, to have his or her hunger satisfied. Babies also have sucking and rooting reflexes that are very well developed at birth. Because of these reflexes, your baby will try to satisfy hunger by rooting and sucking on anything that happens to touch his/her face. Sucking seems to provide comfort to a baby who is hungry or who is simply trying to settle himself/herself. You can meet your baby's need for food and sucking whether you breast or bottle feed. The method you choose is not nearly as important as the nurturing and tender care that takes place while you feed your baby.

BREASTFEEDING

Breastfeeding does provide several advantages to you and your baby. The composition of breast milk is perfectly suited for your infant. Digestion is easier and more complete. Breast fed babies are less likely to develop allergies and have the added benefit of receiving immuno-globulins which provide protection against bacteria and viral infections.

Breast milk is always available and at the right temperature - no need to go to the store to buy it, bring it home, prepare it, and put it into clean bottles. While stored in the breast, it never spoils or gets too old to use.

Breastfeeding also provides advantages to you as a woman. The sucking of the baby at your breast triggers the pituitary gland to release a hormone called oxytocin, a hormone which causes your uterus to contract. Therefore, nursing in the early days helps to minimize bleeding and stimulates the uterus to contract and return to its normal size and shape.

You can expect a few weeks of trial and error, doubts, and fatigue. You may have thoughts of giving bottles of formula so that you are able to tell how much milk your baby has taken. It's best to wait several weeks to give your baby an occasional bottle so that you don't reduce your milk supply. Early, frequent, regular nursing is your best insurance for an adequate milk supply. Rest and drinking fluids are also helpful. Lie down or sit in a rocking chair while you feed your baby. Drink a glass of milk or some other nutritious beverage before or during your nursing.

After your baby is about a month old and this initial learning period is passed, breastfeeding becomes more simple, relaxing and satisfying. You've probably learned by now that your baby will nurse until satisfied and that feedings can be as close as every two hours and as far apart as 4–5 hours. A good rule of thumb to follow is this: your baby is probably getting enough to eat if he/she is feeding every 2–5 hours, has 6 or more wet diapers a day, has frequent bowel movements and sleeps several hours at a time during a 24 hour period.

If your baby is fussy during or after feedings, try soothing the infant by gently rocking or burping. A baby who cries vigorously may have swallowed air or may have a gas bubble from the previous feeding. Always offer the second breast. If your baby is full, he/she will simply stop nursing or refuse the second breast. At the next feeding start the baby nursing on the second breast. A safety pin attached to the bra strap is a good way to remember which breast should be used for the next feeding.

Breast milk is almost always adequate for complete nutrition until a baby is between 4 and 6 months old. By this time, your baby will probably have used up the supply of iron stored during intrauterine development. Iron enriched vitamin drops are frequently prescribed at this time, and foods containing iron can be started.

When to wean your baby from the breast is an individual decision. There is no absolutely ideal time; although, your baby will benefit nutritionally from breast milk if breastfed for the best part of his/her first year of life.

However, you need not justify or defend earlier weaning. When breast feeding no longer meets your or your baby's needs or you simply decide you do not wish to continue, begin slowly to wean to a bottle or a cup. Slow weaning gives you a chance to eliminate gradually one feeding every week or so, giving both you and your baby a chance to adjust. Weaning a child to a bottle will be easier if you have offered your baby a bottle of breast milk or formula at least once a week starting at one month of age. You can start offering sips from a cup when your baby is 5 or 6 months of age.

There are many resources available to the breast feeding family. A local nursing mothers' counselors group and LaLeche League are very helpful organizations whose members can assist you and offer support. There are also a number of good books that give complete "how-to" and "what if" information (see bibliography on page 79).

BOTTLEFEEDING

If you choose to bottle feed your baby, you need to select a nurser set or bottles and nipples. There are many brands and types. You may want to choose nipples that are most like the human breast.

Convenience is also a factor. Some mothers prefer the disposable bottle liners and plastic holders rather than glass bottles. Mothers with access to dishwashers may find glass bottles easier and less expensive to use. Talk to your friends before you buy— experiences of other mothers can be invaluable.

There are various types and brands of commercially prepared formulas which have been produced to closely resemble breast milk. Your doctor can recommend one. It is usually more economical to purchase formula by the case and from a discount store. Ready-made formula may be a life saver the first week or two at home, but it costs much more than liquid concentrate or powdered formula.

When you feed your baby, sit in a comfortable chair or rocker and hold the baby close to you—cradled in your arm. Tilt the bottle so that there is always milk in the nipple to minimize the sucking in of air. Take your time. Talk to and look at your baby. These are precious moments.

Sometimes your baby may gulp down the formula too rapidly to satisfy his/her sucking need. You may want to change to a nipple with a smaller hole or give your baby a pacifier. Don't worry if your baby doesn't empty the bottle. Most babies will stop feeding when their hunger is satisfied.

Bottle fed babies often go longer between feedings than breast fed babies because formula is not digested as rapidly as breast milk. However, most babies will want to eat every two or four hours. Many babies do best if fed on a demand basis rather than a rigid schedule. Every baby is an individual who needs to be fed according to individual needs. He/she may not conform to your expectations. As your baby grows, his/her demands will change. A flexible schedule will provide for these changes and will minimize your baby's fussy periods.

MORE THAN FOOD

Most parents instinctively provide the love and security a baby needs regardless of the method used to feed their baby. As you hold, feed, bathe, dress and play with your baby, you are communicating through touch, sound, and vision. Your baby senses your pleasure with him/her and responds by watching, listening, moving, feeling your touch and trying to talk. It's almost as if you were in synchrony with your baby. When you talk and gaze at your baby, he/she gazes back at you. If you talk, your baby follows the movement of your mouth and may try to imitate you. You have engaged each other by sending messages back and forth to one another. Feeding times are ideal for building this relationship and trust.

When your baby cries and seems hungry, it is natural for him/her to expect to be comforted and fed. As time goes on, you learn how to interpret your baby's cries. You learn to distinguish the frantic, fists-in-the-mouth hunger cry from the whiny fretty cry which often means your baby is over-tired or can't get comfortable.

You may feel frustrated when your baby cries, and you are unable to stop it. Every parent has felt this way at one time or another. It may be reassuring to know that a young baby is not trying to annoy or manipulate you. Your baby has no other way of telling you "I need something." If you respond to your baby by picking him/her up, you are telling your baby, "I know you need something, and I care about you." If you do not respond to your baby's crying because you are afraid of spoiling him/her or because the clock tells you it's not time for a feeding, your baby may learn to cry excessively in order to get you to respond.

A fretty, irritable baby is sometimes difficult to live with. The following tips may help you deal with your baby's fussy times more easily.

COLIC

Colic is sometimes the cause of a crying episode. You can recognize the symptoms if your baby draws his/her knees up in pain, cries very hard and becomes red in the face, or passes gas while crying. Comfort measures you can use for a "colicky" baby are:

1. Walking baby using a baby carrier that holds baby close to your warm body.
2. Holding baby across your lap on his/her abdomen, rocking side to side and gently rubbing back.
3. Laying baby on abdomen next to a hot water bottle wrapped in a towel
4. Provide a pacifier for baby to suck on
5. Minimizing stimulating noise and bright lights
6. Getting relief for yourself by having other family members or friends take turns rocking and soothing baby.

BETWEEN FEEDINGS

Rule out hunger as a cause for your baby's crying. Then consider trying these comfort measures:

1. Touch your baby's neck below his/her hairline in the back. If it feels sweaty, your baby may be too warm. Take off his/her undershirt or remove one layer of clothing. Baby's bedroom need not be warmer than 68°F. In fact, your baby will sleep

and breathe better if the air is not overheated and dry. Add a layer of clothing or a light weight blanket if your baby's neck feels cool. (Baby's hands and feet are usually cool to the touch and are not good indicators of the baby's temperature.)

2. Change your baby's position. Tiny babies are most comfortable lying on their abdomen. This position feels safe because it gives a sense of balance and gives baby a chance to tuck his/her legs up under the abdomen.

3. Move your baby to a different room. Give him/her a change of scenery. Some babies enjoy being near other people and around activities. Use a safe infant seat so your baby can see what's going on.

4. Sing to your baby, or play music on the radio, record player or musical toy.

5. Help your baby adjust to your home and lifestyle by being natural. There is no need to tiptoe, whisper, or avoid making normal noises. Babies are amazingly adaptable and soon learn to select or tune out certain sounds.

6. Try using a baby carrier, swing, rocker, stroller or a ride in a car. Babies respond to motion because they are accustomed to the gentle movement of their mother's body during pregnancy. Babies need cuddling and holding—it's reassuring to them.

7. Take your baby for a walk outside if weather permits. Fresh air can be refreshing and may provide enough stimulation to overcome the boredom of looking at the same walls and toys. Babies often nap especially well after an outing.

OVERSTIMULATION

There are times when despite your most sincere efforts, it is impossible to soothe a crying baby. Trust your instincts and feelings in this matter. When you feel you have done all you are willing or capable of doing, or when you feel the baby may be overstimulated, then it's time to put the baby in its crib. Once you have done this, leave the baby in the crib even if he/she continues to cry for 10 or 15 minutes. Offer the baby a pacifier. Gently pat his/her bottom. If this doesn't work, simply leave the room; close the door; and busy yourself with something else. If necessary to calm yourself, sit in the yard or turn on music or TV softly to help yourself relax.

It is not necessary to respond 100% of your time to your baby's needs. The important thing to remember is that as a parent, you know what is best for your child most of the time. As time goes on, you will learn and grow in your parenting. Each day will provide additional experiences. You'll learn what works and what doesn't work, what feels good and what doesn't feel good. You'll also learn that it takes time to become the parent you are capable of being.

As long as you respond to your baby in a positive and loving way, the baby will learn to trust you and to think of this world as a good place to be. Parents and baby will also feel a strong attachment to one another which helps cushion the tense or difficult times which are a normal part of every family's development.

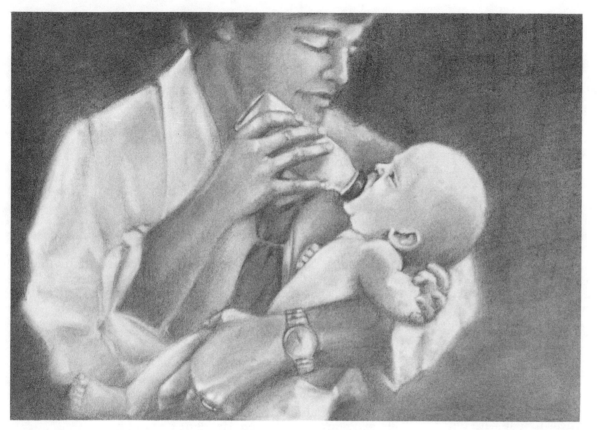

REALITIES OF EARLY PARENTING

For quite some time now, the focus of your attention has been on "getting through the labor and delivery." It may be almost too frightening and overwhelming to think about what your life will be like once you and your baby are home and begin a new life as a family. Sometimes the reality of being parents hits you when you get home that first day from the hospital. You realize there is no turning back.

Probably, some confidence in caretaking ability has been established by both parents as the result of early contact with your baby while you were in the hospital. However, you are both still learning—learning to physically care for your baby, learning what to do when he or she cries or perhaps learning to breastfeed. It can be frustrating to be unsure of the many questions and problems that arise in the first months of an infant's life, such

as: "Why is he crying? What are we doing wrong? Will we spoil him if we pick him up every time he cries?"

Time, practice and patience will gradually provide the answers to these and many other questions. So will a good book or two on child care and a good pediatrician or family doctor. However, the real challenge is coping with the feelings and conflict new parenthood can bring. The basic theme is usually this: the baby completely disrupts the couple's lives, and they each experience a sense of loss. There is the loss of freedom—time and ability to choose recreation, to express affection spontaneously, to get work done and to be alone. There is the loss of companionship and even the loss of individuality as each of you begins to define his or her role as mother or father, rather than your individual personality.

All too often these feelings surface as jealousy toward the infant, when a more accurate and realistic explanation would be resentment and anxiety about the "losses" you are experiencing.

For example, consider the following specific issues that in many instances have to be dealt with during the early months of parenting.

1. FATIGUE

A woman may automatically expect her spouse to realize how tired she feels and assume that he will automatically help with the baby and housework. But the only time she tells him how tired she is occurs when she's angry at him or when refusing sexual advances. He only hears the attack on him, not her plea for help, and reacts accordingly. At the same time, he may be experiencing problems at work and the strains of having an infant at home are fatiguing to him, too. He needs a few minutes of relaxation before he can give the help he is probably quite willing to give. But he too expresses his fatigue when defending himself against complaints. Only by honestly confronting the problem of fatigue can you change work load, experiment with different solutions and change them as the need arises.

2. HELP WITH INFANT CARE

What appears to be the father's unwillingness to help with the baby is seen by the new mother as a sign of laziness, sexism and lack of love for her and the baby. Even though she is overtired, she may not be willing to give up the caretaking responsibilities to the baby's father. He may be afraid of doing the wrong thing. Her impatience and her own anxieties will only make him feel incompetent and worthless. Much of this conflict can be avoided by sharing in the baby's care as soon as possible after birth. Then, both parents can provide mutual help and support; share tips they learn and gain confidence and expertise from each other.

3. LOVE, AFFECTION AND SEX

These areas can be the touchiest of all and the most difficult to express. Problems with your sex life can undermine your closeness as a couple at a time when your closeness is threatened in many other ways as well. Tension and conflict about resuming intercourse, as well as physical adjustments—episiotomy, lack of natural lubrication, leaking of milk from the breasts—all add to the awkwardness one may feel when it comes to sexual intercourse.

A new mother may resist affection from her mate for fear it will lead to intercourse which she may not always want. She may even be hesitant to kiss or hug or let him show affection toward her unless she wants intercourse. Conversely, he may see her stiffening whenever he caresses her and take it as a sign of rejection. He may also misinterpret her lack of willingness for intercourse as lack of love.

If the baby sleeps in the same bedroom, both parents may be distracted by the baby's noises or embarrassed about having intercourse. It is common for a woman who has recently given birth to be self conscious about her flabby stomach, or the slowly fading stretch marks and her sensitive breasts. She may even feel that her body is no longer her own property but is being claimed by both baby and husband.

The father may feel all of this is a sign that her body is now forbidden territory to all but the baby and that he has been replaced. He assumes this because she doesn't say anything about being tense or embarrassed. He won't take the risk of admitting he feels awkward and is even afraid of hurting her.

So each partner is left to guess what the other is thinking, and it is almost always a negative guess. Consequently, they avoid the very expression of affection that each needs very much.

To help you ease through this adjustment period, use a lubricant such as KY or Lubrifax to moisten the vaginal area. Try to be sure the baby is asleep and in another room before you begin lovemaking. Respect each other's feelings about when to have intercourse. Once you start having relations, don't give up if you run into problems. Talk openly about them and help each other to understand. Gain perspective from the other's point of view.

Fatigue, help with infant care, companionship, love, affection and sex, although discussed separately, are interrelated. The solutions to any one of them often helps to solve others. By early and consistent "partnering" in caretaking and chores, both partners have more time to be individuals with each other. Avoid thinking of the father's time spent with his child as "babysitting." His contribution to child raising is as equally important as the mother's—time spent in child care can never be construed as babysitting.

4. COMPANIONSHIP

Very frequently a mother feels starved for companionship and adult conversation. She can hardly wait for her mate to come home and is hurt if he doesn't confide in her any more about his work, doesn't chat with her or doesn't seem to see her as a person. She may not realize that she is engrossed in the baby and that her first words when he returns home are a demand for help. Her questions about work are often superficial and she doesn't realize her mate needs a short time to regroup himself before he is capable of "pitching in."

The father, on the other hand, doesn't realize that what he sees as "protecting" her from his own worries is actually shutting her out of an important part of his life. He, too, may sorely miss the companionship they had formerly given each other and is just as hurt as she is. Honest comparison of each other's need for companionship can clear up misinterpretations and find solutions.

A time to relax and chat together as a couple provides more companionship and recreation. Set a pattern of going out together as early as possible postpartum. Being away from your baby for brief periods of time can do much to help you regain your sense of pleasure with each other and help you relax and enjoy your baby more.

Not all problems have solutions. No amount of communication and understanding can find time that isn't there, or will change a relationship back to the way it was before the baby was born, or remove all the hassles of infant care. They have to work themselves out in time or through counseling with your physician, mental health clinic or family therapist. If you would like to share your feelings with other parents, join a group such as Family Centered Parents; Post Partum: "Mothers Are People Too;" STEP (Systematic Training for Effective Parenting).

To help prepare yourselves for parenting and realize your expectations of each other as parents, complete and discuss the family contract found on the following pages.

FAMILY CONTRACT

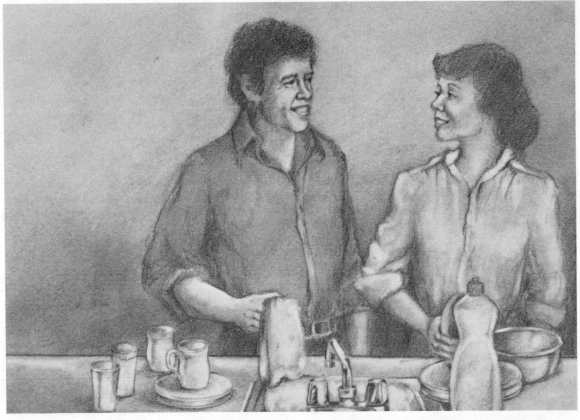

Within a family structure there is usually some separation of responsibility, depending upon cultural backgrounds, life style and the personal abilities of each family member. It is important that these responsibilities be shared so personal exploitation of any individual does not result from the breakdown of whose job it is to do what.

Much conflict and resentment can be avoided if family members understand and appreciate each other's expectations and are willing to "cross-train" each other so each will be able to take over the responsibilities of the other if the need arises. If children grow up in the kind of family environment that allows this flexibility, they will have the opportunity to identify with parents who can move freely among all the assignments whose completion is necessary for the maintenance of a healthy family life.

The children in a family with a fair and equitable "contract" will not associate any one role with either masculinity or femininity—they will see both parents as equally important caretakers of the home and the children.

This chart is a good example of the kinds of responsibilities involved in homemaking and childbearing. Look at each of the following tasks and ask yourself, "Whose responsibility is this?" Then select the number which represents your answer. The lower numbers reflect the father's responsibility, the higher numbers reflect the mother's responsibility. Numbers in the middle range reflect the opinion that the task is the responsibility of both.

Even if both agree that certain tasks are the total responsibility of the father or mother, harmony will result. It is the areas of wide disagreement that are most likely to cause some resentment and disharmony. These are the ones you will need to work through, although it is unlikely you will always agree on everything.

FATHER'S RESPONSIBILITY				BOTH			MOTHER'S RESPONSIBILITY	
1	2	3	4	5	6	7	8	9

HER OPINION	HIS OPINION	GENERAL AREAS	HER OPINION	HIS OPINION	CHILD CARE
____	____	planning and preparing meals	____	____	feeding
____	____	cleaning up after meals	____	____	reading to, playing with
____	____	repairs around the house	____	____	health care (doctor, dentist) appointments
____	____	house cleaning			
____	____	shopping	____	____	transporting to and from child care
____	____	paying bills	____	____	getting ready for bed
____	____	washing and ironing	____	____	rocking, soothing, holding
____	____	making social arrangements	____	____	caring for sick child
____	____	looking after the car	____	____	getting up at night when baby cries
____	____	providing family income	____	____	diapering
____	____	home decorating	____	____	toilet training
____	____	mowing lawn, shoveling snow	____	____	staying home from work when baby is sick
____	____	weeding, garden, flowers			
____	____	outside painting			
____	____	birth control			

GUIDE TO PREVENTION OF PREGNANCY

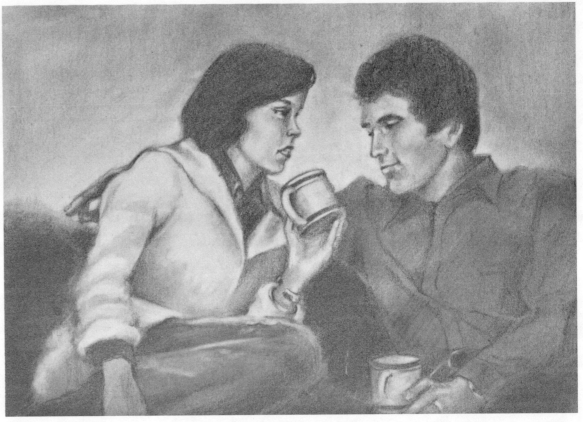

Wanted babies are usually happy babies. Over 80% of sexually active people use some sort of birth control to prevent pregnancy. Sometimes birth control is used to delay or space children.

Birth control is a personal matter largely determined by your lifestyle, age, religion, state of health and your knowledge about methods of contraception. Talk to someone who is knowledgeable about birth control—your family physician or obstetrician, health workers in planned parenthood clinic or the gynecology clinic in a hospital.

After reading this guide about various methods to prevent pregnancy, you will know the current available methods, how they are used and their extent of reliability.

More detailed information can then be obtained, or an acceptable method prescribed, fitted or applied by a physician. If pos-

sible, both partners should be involved in the decision in choosing an acceptable method to birth control. It may be helpful to take this guide with you to the doctor or clinic. Ask questions and seek additional information until you feel you are adequately informed and prepared.

Generally speaking, pregnancy is prevented by interfering with the union of the ovum (egg) and sperm or by preventing the fertilized egg from attaching itself to the lining of the uterus. Different methods may be used at different times in your life. A method that is acceptable and right for you now, may not be the method you will use five years from now.

There are six major reliable methods for the control of conception: oral tablets, intrauterine devices (IUD), vaginal spermicides, vaginal diaphragm with spermicide, natural family planning, and voluntary sterilization.

ORAL TABLETS (Birth Control Pills)

These small tablets contain estrogen and progesterone (pregnancy hormones) which halt ovulation. They must be prescribed by a physician. One tablet is taken daily for 21 or 28 consecutive days each month. It is not uncommon for women to experience signs of early pregnancy the first few months while taking oral contraceptives. These symptoms usually lessen with each month as the body adjusts to the hormone levels.

It is important that a woman taking an oral contraceptive notify her physician whenever any of the following conditions occur:

Frequent or persistent headaches.

Discoloration of skin.

Unexplained pains in the chest.

Unusual swelling of the ankles.

Shortness of breath.

Some disturbance in vision, such as "seeing double" or sudden partial or complete loss of sight.

Unusual, persistent or unexplained pain in the legs.

Lumps or growths on the breast.

Frequent or persistent vaginal bleeding.

Oral contraceptives are extremely effective if taken correctly. However, there is an increased risk of heart attack and stroke to women who smoke while taking birth control pills. Also, some women who have taken birth control pills while they are breastfeeding find that their milk supply is definitely reduced. Because of the effects and possible hazards of hormone drugs on breastfed babies, mothers should use another type of contraceptive while nursing.

INTRAUTERINE DEVICE (IUD)

This contraceptive device is usually cylindrically shaped plastic or variously shaped metal. The physician straightens the device and inserts it with a small applicator into the cavity of the uterus. After being placed into the uterine cavity, it returns to its original shape and usually remains there indefinitely, depending on the type of device. It is thought that the device prevents the fertilized egg from attaching itself to the lining of the uterus.

Several types of IUD's must be removed and a new one reinserted periodically. A small percentage of women reject the device, in which case it is partially or totally passed out of the uterus. There is also a slight risk that the device may perforate the uterus and cause serious complications.

The IUD is a relatively safe method of birth control and is almost as effective as oral contraceptive tablets.

VAGINAL SPERMICIDES

Spermicides are substances containing chemicals that will kill sperm without harming vaginal tissue. These products are available in four forms—foam, cream, jelly and suppositories. With the exception of the suppository, all are applied with thin plastic applicators. Only one application is required before each act of intercourse, and they are significantly more effective than rhythm, withdrawal, condom or so called "hygiene" suppositories or douching.

Most can be obtained without a prescription. A new spermicide in the form of a vaginal suppository has recently been developed and, if used properly, is quite effective.

VAGINAL DIAPHRAGMS WITH SPERMICIDES

The diaphragm is a strong round rubber disc about the size of a medium sized jar lid. The rim of the diaphragm is a flexible rubber covered metal spring which bends so that it can be compressed and inserted into the vagina. After being inserted into the uppermost part of the vagina, it opens to form a cap over the cervix.

Each woman must be properly fitted for a diaphragm by a physician. When properly fitted and covered with a spermicidal jelly or cream, the diaphragm acts as a barrier, preventing sperm from entering the uterus; and the spermicide kills the sperm. This method of birth control is very effective. Many women use the diaphragm and spermicide together because it is a visible means of two-fold protection against pregnancy.

NATURAL FAMILY PLANNING

The natural method of family planning avoid the use of chemical or artificial means of preventing pregnancy. Instead, daily observations of signs and symptoms which normally occur in every woman's menstrual cycle are used.

There are four basic types of natural family planning methods: The Ovulation Method (sometimes referred to as the Billings Method), the Basal Body Temperature Method, the Sympto-Thermal Method and the Calendar Rhythm Method.

The Ovulation Method

This method of natural family planning teaches a woman how to test and interpret her vaginal secretions which change during her menstrual cycle. Immediately following a menstrual period, no mucus is seen or felt. As the cycle continues, a yellow or white thick mucus is secreted by the crevix. This mucus feels sticky to the touch. As the ovary is about to release an ovum, the estrogen stimulation changes the mucus to a clear, slippery substance which feels and looks like raw egg white. After ovulation, the mucous decreases and becomes sticky again.

The success of this method is dependent upon the couple's abstaining from intercourse during the time the mucus is slippery and wet, plus approximately 72 hours following this time. It is a useful method for women who are breastfeeding and for women who have irregular cycles.

The Basal Body Temperature Method

The temperature method depends on the day-to-day taking and recording of the basal body temperature (BBT). The time of ovulation can be identified when there is a rise in the BBT as a result of an increase in the level of progesterone. The BBT is most helpful in determining when the post-ovulatory infertile phase takes place.

The Sympto-Thermal Method

As the name implies, symptoms of ovulation as well as temperature changes are observed and used to determine when ovulation occurs. Other signs and symptoms of ovulation are also noted, such as abdominal discomfort, spotting, breast sensitivity and mood changes. By combining the ovulation and BBT methods, the natural signs of fertility in a woman's body can guide the couple in planning or avoiding a pregnancy.

The Rhythm Method

Sometimes called the calendar or calendar rhythm, this method relies on a careful calendar record of a woman's menstrual cycles. After observing approximately six months of cycles, an average cycle length can be predicted. However, women with irregular cycles will find this method less than reliable.

Natural Family Planning is available through various clinics, hospitals and organizations. See page 78 for addresses of several such centers.

VOLUNTARY STERILIZATION

Sterilization is a permanent method of birth control for men or women who want no children or who have all the children they desire. It is a surgical procedure that involves the closing of the tubes that carry the sperm or the ovum (egg) so the egg and sperm cannot meet and result in pregnancy. It does not involve removing any reproductive glands—ovaries or testicles—and is not the same as castration.

Tubal sterilization in women can be performed in a number of ways with several types of surgical instruments. Tubal ligation is done by making an incision through the abdomen to cut and close the fallopian tubes. Another frequently used technique is laparoscopy (a tube containing a telescope and light). After a harmless gas is used to distend the abdomen for better visibility, the laparoscope and an instrument to seal the tubes are passed through one or two small incisions below the navel. After the instruments are removed and the gas released, the incisions are covered with bandaids. Sometimes this is called a tubal coagulation.

There are several other types of less commonly known methods of tubal sterilization: mini-laparotomy, colpotomy and culdoscopy. Information on these methods can be obtained from your physician or planned parenthood clinic.

Tubal ligation performed through an abdominal incision requires general anesthesia and a hospital stay from three to five days. A laparoscopic tubal coagulation may be done under general or local anesthesia and usually only requires an overnight or less than 24 hour hospital stay.

All surgery carries some risk—bleeding, infection, trauma to other organs, risk from anesthetic agents, etc. However, such serious problems happen in only a small number of cases. Be sure to discuss both risks and benefits with your physician before reaching a decision.

Sterilization for a man, called vasectomy, is minor surgery and is usually performed in the physician's office or clinic under local anesthesia. The physician makes one or two incisions in the scrotum through which each sperm-carrying tube, called the vas deferens, is lifted out, cut and closed, thus blocking the passage of sperm. A man continues to have an erection and ejaculate but the semen (fluid) contains no sperm.

For some time after the operation, sperm already present in the semen and tubes may fertilize the ovum; therefore a contraceptive must be used until tests show sperm are no longer present in the ejaculation.

The risk associated with a vasectomy is smaller than for female sterilization. There is usually some discomfort when the local anesthetic wears off, and swelling and bruising of the scrotal skin. Complications such as hemorrhage, infection, inflammation of the epididymis and sperm granuloma are rare but must be explained before surgery is performed.

Surgical sterilization of either sex should be considered as permanent. There is very low risk of failure in both men and women. To minimize the risk for men, it is very important that they return to the doctor for checkups after a vasectomy to determine when sterility has been achieved. Unfortunately, the only sign of failure in women is a pregnancy.

Your decision to have a sterilization should be made after careful consideration and discussion with your physician and partner. Then decide which one will have the operation, you or your partner. The person who most firmly favors permanent sterilization is the best candidate for the surgery.

Sterilization is not the answer to emotional, marital or sexual problems. But, it can bring you peace of mind and relief from fear of unwanted pregnancy.

LESS THAN RELIABLE METHODS

There are two widely practiced but very unreliable methods of preventing pregnancy. These are the condom and withdrawal.

THE CONDOM

The condom is a thin rubber sheath that is pulled over the penis prior to intercourse. Although sperm is supposed to remain in the sheath, it may slip off or tear during intercourse. If used in conjunction with a spermicidal jelly or cream, this two-fold method provides a relatively greater protection than just using a condom alone.

WITHDRAWAL

Also called coitus interruptus, withdrawal requires a man to withdraw from the vagina just before ejaculation. The weaknesses of this method are several. First of all, sperm is usually present in the lubricating fluids that are secreted from the penis before ejaculation. Only one sperm is needed to fertilize the ovum, so pregnancy can occur despite withdrawal of the penis before ejaculation.

Considerable discipline and experience is required to withdraw completely not only from the internal vagina, but from the external genitalia as well. Many men find this extremely difficult.

The following methods are **not** effective and should not be relied upon to prevent pregnancy: douches, "hygiene" suppositories, capsules, liquids or other substances labeled for "cleanliness or hygiene" use. These products do not contain spermicides or chemicals that destroy sperm on contact. The physical washing of the vaginal canal is not effective since many sperm enter the uterus through the cervix immediately after intercourse. Recent truth in advertising laws makes it more difficult for manufacturers to mislead the public with the use of these products as contraceptives.

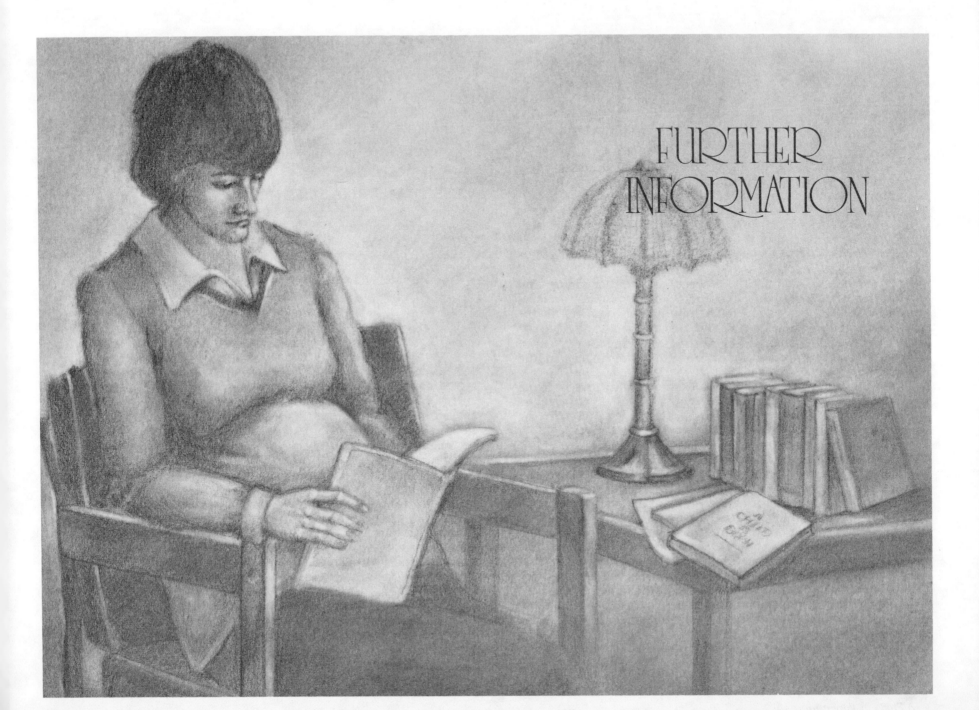

Part IV: Further Information

    A. Terminology and Definitions

    B. Programs and Organizations for Expectant and New Parents

    C. Suggestions for Further Reading

TERMINOLOGY & DEFINITIONS

Understanding some of the medical jargon associated with childbirth will help you when reading this manual and may "demystify" the subject when you discuss childbirth with your doctor, nurse and family.

Even your children can learn the proper names of body parts if you use these terms in conversations with them. Naturally, not all of the terms will become common household words, but you will feel much more comfortable when you hear them if you understand what they mean.

They are listed here alphabetically for easy referral.

1. Apgar: A rating or score given to a newborn at 1 and 5 minutes after birth in regard to color, cry, muscle tone, respirations and reflexes, 0 to 2 points for each one.

2. Braxton Hicks Contractions: Painless, intermittant uterine contractions occurring periodically during pregnancy, thereby enlarging the uterus to accomodate the growing fetus. Become more frequent toward the end of pregnancy and sometimes present a picture of false labor.

3. Bulging: The pushing out and swelling of the vulva, perineum and rectum, due to pressure of the presenting part, a sign that delivery is imminent.

4. Caput: Appearance of the infant's head at the vaginal orifice; also the swelling of the baby's scalp during labor.

5. Cervix: The neck or lower part of the uterus, which dilates and effaces during labor to allow passage of the fetus.

6. Crowning: Appearance of the top of the infant's head at the vaginal orifice so that the vulva "crown" the head as it is ready to pass out of the vagina.

7. Dilatation: Indicates the diameter of the cervical opening and is measured in centimeters, ten centimeters being fully dilated; or in fingers, 2 cms = one finger.

8. E.D.C./E.D.D.: Expected Date of Confinement/Expected Date of Delivery or due date. Found by adding 7 days to the first day of the last menstrual period, and subtracting 3 months.

9. Effacement: Gradual thinning, shortening and drawing up of the cervix. Measured in percentage, 100% being totally effaced, obliteration of cervical canal.

10. Embryo: The name given to the fertilized ovum from the time of fertilization until 8 weeks of gestation.

11. Episiotomy: Surgical incision of the perineum which enlarges the vaginal opening and permits easier delivery.

12. Fetus: The name given to the fertilized ovum after the first 8 weeks of gestation until birth.

13. F.H.T.: F.H.R.: Fetal Heart Tones or Rate. First heard at about 20 weeks gestation. Normal rate is 120-160 beats a minute.

14. Fundus: The upper rounded portion of the uterus.

15. Gravida: Number of pregnancies.

16. Lightening: The sensation of decreased abdominal pressure produced by the descent of the uterus into the pelvic cavity, which usually occurs prior to the onset of labor.

17. Lochia: The discharge of blood, mucus and tissue from the uterus during the 6 week period following delivery (puerperium).

18. Membranes: The bag of waters, whose principle purpose is to protect the fetus from trauma and infection and to provide the fetus freedom of movement and constant temperature.

19. Multipara: (Multip) A woman who has had or is giving birth to her second or more child.

20. Para: Past pregnancies which have produced an infant of 28 weeks or more gestation, stillborn or alive.

21. Perineum: The area between the vagina and rectum.

22. Phases of First Stage of Labor: Early: 0-4 centimeters dilatation
Middle: 4-8 centimeters
Transition: 8-10 centimeters

23. Placenta: The circular, flat organ in the pregnant uterus which serves as the exchange station for nourishment and elimination of wastes. Also known as afterbirth.

24. Premature Infant: An infant weighing less than 2,500 Gms or 5 lbs., 8 oz. at birth, or born before 37 weeks gestation.

25. Primagravida: (Primip) A woman who is pregnant for the first time.

26. Primapara: (Primip) A woman who has had or is giving birth to her first child.

27. Quickening: The mother's first perception of the movements of the fetus.

28. Show: Blood-tinged mucus discharge from the vagina before and during labor.

29. Stages of Labor: First: From the onset of labor contractions to complete dilatation and effacement of the cervix— 0-10 centimeters.
Second: From the complete dilatation and effacement of the cervix to birth of the infant.
Third: From the birth of the infant to the delivery of the placenta (afterbirth).

30. Station: Indicates the position of the fetus in the pelvis by describing the relation of the presenting part of the fetus (usually the head) to the isheal spines of the pelvis. Measured in centimeters—how far the part is above or below the spines. If above the spines, it is -1, -2, -3 and floating; if below the spines, it is +1, +2, +3 and on the perineum; if level with the spines, it is at 'zero station'.

31. Toxemia: A disease of pregnancy manifested by high blood pressure, protein in the urine and swelling; most always found in the last three months of pregnancy. Cause unknown.

32. Uterus: The pear shaped muscular organ that houses the fetus, placenta, amniotic fluid and other products of conception. Sometimes referred to as "womb" it greatly increases in size and capacity during pregnancy.

PROGRAMS & ORGANIZATIONS FOR EXPECTANT & NEW PARENTS

Some agencies, programs and support groups are available both locally and nationwide. Frequently, new parents are isolated from family or have recently moved to a new area and have not had time to cultivate new friends and support systems.

The following is a partial listing of organizations which will help expectant and new parents better cope with the many aspects of childbearing and child raising.

PARENT INFORMATION

Action for Child Transportation Safety (ACTS)
400 Central Park West, 15P
New York, New York 10025

This organization is devoted to educating parents about child automobile safety. Send a stamped, self-addressed envelope for a booklet and fact sheet.

Allergy Foundation of America
801 Second Avenue
New York, New York 10017

This group has a number of booklets on childhood allergies. Send stamped, self-addressed envelope for information.

American Academy of Pediatrics
1801 Hinman Avenue
Evanston, Illinois 60204

This medical organization, made up of most of the nation's practicing pediatricians, has compiled information for parents on safety, immunizations, and health care of children. Send stamped, self-addressed envelope.

American National Red Cross
17 & D Streets
Washington, D.C. 20006

Address inquiries to Nursing Department to obtain information on Red Cross classes on baby care, prenatal care, adoptive parenting, and family living.
Local Red Cross Chapter: Address
                          Phone No.

Birthright
62 Hunter Street
Woodbury, New Jersey 08096
Phone No. (609) 848-1818

Birthright is a pro-life pregnancy counseling service which offers positive alternatives to abortion. It is staffed by trained volunteers and operates on financial donations from individuals and organizations. Birthright is independent, non-political, non-sectarian and prepared to help women, whether single or married, regardless of age, race, or religion. This service is free, confidential and non-judgemental.
Local Birthright: Address
                   Phone No.

C/Sec., Inc.
Cesarean/Support Education and Concern
15 Maynard Road
Dedham, MA 02026

This non-profit organization is committed to improving the cesarean birth experience. Local cesarean birth support groups are being formed; some are official branches of this national organization.
Local Cesarean Birth Support Group: Name
                                     Address
                                     Phone No.

LaLeche League
9616 Minneapolis Avenue
Franklin Park, Illinois 10605

An organization which promotes information and assistance to breastfeeding families. Monthly meetings are held in the form of a four part sequence of programs for nursing mothers and are usually held in homes of League leaders.
Local LaLeche Chapter or Leader: Name
                                  Address
                                  Phone No.

Another source for breastfeeding information is a group of volunteers such as Nursing Mothers Counselors who provide counseling and non-medical advice and information. Some hospitals provide this service and may have a NMC visit mothers in the hospital and teach classes on breastfeeding.

National Foundation - March of Dimes
1275 Mamaroneck Avenue
White Plains, New York 10605

This organization is devoted to preventing and curing birth defects. Many booklets, films, and film strips are available to the public and can be obtained by writing or calling the national or local chapter.

National Organization of Mothers of Twins Clubs
5402 Amberwood Lane
Rockville, Maryland 20853

Through this organization, you can learn of local chapters and share interests and concerns with other mothers of twins.

CHILDBIRTH EDUCATION ORGANIZATIONS AND INSTRUCTORS

American Academy of Husband Coached Childbirth
(also called the Bradley Method)
P.O. Box 5224
Sherman Oaks, CA 91413

An organization which promotes the Bradley method of prepared childbirth and provides training and certification of teachers.

The Bradley method endorses true natural childbirth by using complete deep relaxation, the natural sleeping position and deep diaphragmatic breathing during labor.

Local Bradley Method Instructor: Name
                                 Address
                                 Phone No.

American Society for Psychoprophylaxis in Obstetrics (ASPO) (commonly referred to as Lamaze)
1411 K Street, Northwest
Washington, D.C. 20005
Phone No. (202) 783-7050

A non-profit educational organization aimed at meeting the ever-increasing demand of American women for precise information and training in childbirth. ASPO is composed of three divisions—physicians, teachers, and parents—with a nine member board of directors consisting of three elected representatives from each division. ASPO maintains an information and referral service designed to help women obtain training. Names of member teachers and physicians are given to expectant mothers upon request. In addition, the Society supplies the necessary teaching materials, maintains a film rental and reference library, and sponsors teacher training courses open to qualified nurses and physical therapists.

Local ASPO Certified Instructor: Name
                                 Address
                                 Phone No.

International Childbirth Education Association (ICEA)

The purpose of this organization is to join together groups and individuals to more actively and effectively further the preparation of expectant parents for childbirth; enhance parent-child relationships by encouraging breastfeeding; encourage, guide, and set standards for training programs for childbirth; work with health care systems in furthering parent participation and minimal obstetric intervention in uncomplicated labors; further the study and application of knowledge concerning family-centered maternity and child care; and further a wider understanding and acceptance of these aims among health professionals and lay people.

There are many ICEA member groups, individual members and ICEA recognized teacher training centers.

ICEA
P. O. Box 20048
Minneapolis, Minnesota 55420

Local ICEA Group or Instructor: Name
                                     Address
                                     Phone No.

The American Foundation for Maternal
  and Child Health
30 Beekman Place
New York, NY 10022
Phone Number (212) 759-5510

PARENTING PROGRAMS AND ORGANIZATIONS

Numerous programs on the national, state, and local level are available. Many are "packaged" or structured programs and others are developed through schools, hospitals, mental health agencies and childbirth education groups. Examples of such programs are:

Parent Effectiveness Training (PET)

Systematic Training for Effective Parenting (STEP)

Early Childhood Development

ICEA Parenting Programs

Parents Anonymous (for abusive parents)

Parents Without Partners (for single parents)

Parent-Teacher Associations or Organizations (PTA or PTO)

ASPO Parenting Programs

"Mothers Are People, Too" (Postpartum Support Group)

U.S. Consumer Product Safety Commission
Washington, D.C. 20207
Phone No. (800) 492-2937

By calling this toll free number, you can obtain information on safety standards for cribs, toys and other accessories for children. Many booklets are also available upon request.

NATURAL FAMILY PLANNING ORGANIZATIONS

The Couple to Couple League
P. O. Box 11084
Cincinnati, Ohio 45211
Phone No. (513) 661-7612

The Human Life Center
St. John's University
Collegeville, Minnesota 56321

The Natural Family Planning Federation
1511 "K" Street, N. W.
Washington, DC 20005

SUGGESTIONS FOR FURTHER READING

There are many—probably hundreds—of books on pregnancy, childbirth, child care, parenting and breast feeding. And there are almost as many opinions and controversies among authors. The following bibliography lists some of the most recent and informative books available in bookstores, libraries and from mail order suppliers. This listing is by no means complete nor is it meant to be. This bibliography will help you to select several works from the large number of books currently on the market.

PREGNANCY, PRENATAL DEVELOPMENT, PREPARING FOR PARENTHOOD

1. *A Child Is Born*, Nilsson, Lennart, et al. New York: Delacorte Press, 1977.

2. *A Guide to Pregnancy and Parenthood for Women on Their Own*, Ashdown-Sharp, Patricia. New York: Vintage Books, 1977.

3. *Baby Dance—A Comprehensive Guide to Prenatal and Postpartum Exercise*, Markoivitz, Elysa and Brainen, Howard, Englewood Cliffs, New Jersey: Prentice Hall, Inc. 1980.

4. *Caring For Your Unborn Child*, Gots, Ronald and Gots, Barbara, New York: Bantam Books, 1977.

5. *Making Love During Pregnancy*, Bing, Elizabeth and Colman, Libby. 1977.

6. *Pregnancy After 35*, McCauley, Carole, Spearin. New York: E.P. Dutton & Co., Inc., 1976.

7. *Teenage Pregnancy: A New Beginning*, Barr, Linda and Monserrat, Catherine. Albuquerque: New Futures, Inc., 1978.

8. *The Child Before Birth*, Annis, Linda. Ithica, Cornell University Press, 1978.

9. *The Expectant Father*, Schaefer, George, M.D., New York: Barnes & Noble Books, 1972.

10. *The Rights of the Pregnant Parent*, Elkins, V. New York: Two Continents Publishing Group, 1976.

11. *What Every Pregnant Woman Should Know: The Truth About Diets and Drugs In Pregnancy*, Brewer, Gail and Tom. New York: Random House, 1977.

LABOR AND DELIVERY, PREPARATION FOR CHILDBIRTH

1. *Birth Without Violence*, LeBoyer, Dr. Frederick. New York: Alfred A. Knopf, 1975.

2. *Cesarean Birth Experience*, Donovan, Bonnie. Boston: Beacon Press, 1977.

3. *Cesarean Celebration*, Vestal, Laurie. Middleton, WI; EM Printers, 1978.

4. *Childbirth Without Fear*, Dick-Read, Grantly, M.D. New York: Harper & Row Publishers, 1970.

5. *Have It Your Way*, Walton, Vicki E. Seattle: Henry Philips Publishing Company, 1977.

6. *Methods of Childbirth*, Bean, Constance, New York: Dolphin Books (Doubleday & Co., Inc.) 1974.

7. *Six Practical Lessons for an Easier Childbirth*, Bing, Elizabeth. New York: Bantam, 1977.

8. *Choices in Childbirth*, Feldman, Silvia. New York: Grosset & Dunlap, 1978.

BREASTFEEDING

1. *Nursing Your Baby*, Prior, Karen. New York: Harper & Row Publishers, 1963.

2. *Preparation for Breastfeeding*, Ewy, Donna & Rodger. Garden City, New York: Doubleday, Co. 1975.

3. *The Complete Book of Breastfeeding*, Eiger, Marvin and Olds, Sally. New York: Bantam Books, 1973.

4. *The Womanly Art of Breastfeeding*, LaLeche League International: Franklin Park, Illinois, 1963.

INFANT AND CHILD CARE; THE ART OF BEING A PARENT

1. *Baby and Child Care,* Spock, Benjamin. New York: Pocket Books, Inc., 1966.

2. *Between Parent and Child,* Ginott, Dr. Haim. New York: Avon Books, 1965.

3. *Raising the Only Child,* Kappelman, Murray. New York: New American Library, 1975.

4. *Teenage Parents,* Edwards, Margot. Seattle: Pennypress, 1978.

5. *The First Three Years of Life,* White, Burton, Englewood Cliffs, New Jersey: Prentice Hall, Inc. 1975.

6. *What Every Child Would Like His Parents to Know,* Salk, Dr. Lee. New York: Warner Paperback Library, 1973.

7. *Your Child from 1 to 12,* Salk, Dr. Lee. New York: New American Library, Inc., 1970.

8. *The Roots of Love,* Arnstein, Helene. New York: Bantam Books, Inc., 1977.

PREPARING SIBLINGS FOR BIRTH OF THE BABY

1. *A New Baby At Our House,* Martin, Gilbert. New York: Grosset & Dunlap, 1980.

2. *How Was I Born?* Nilsson, Lennart. New York: Dial-Delacorte, 1975.

3. *The Wonderful Story of How You Were Born,* Gruenberg, Sidonie. New York: Doubleday & Co., Inc. 1970.

4. *Where Do Babies Come From?* (Famous award winning B.B.C. program adapted for reading) Sheffield, Margaret. New York: Alfred A. Knopf, Inc., 1972.

POSTPARTUM

1. *Help for Depressed Mothers,* Ciaramitaro, Barbara. Talent, Oregon: 1978.

2. *The Growth and Development of Mothers,* McBride, Angela. New York: Harper & Row, 1973.

3. *The Joy of Being A Woman,* Trobisch, Ingred. New York: Harper & Row, 1975.

4. *The Mother Person,* Barber, Virginia and Skaggs, Merrill. New York: Schocken Books, Inc., 1973.

5. *What Now? A Handbook for New Parents,* Rozdilsky & Banat. New York: Charles Scribner's Sons, 1975.

S0-DMY-061

Missing!

By Dawn McMillan

Illustrated by Julian Bruere

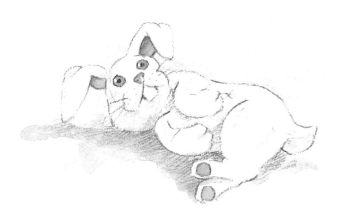

Rocky Meets Devon and Rabbit

Jason tapped his foot, and Rocky came running through the living room and into the kitchen.

"Look at him!" laughed Danny. "He knows his way around the furniture already!"

Jason patted his puppy and signed to Danny, "He's clever!"

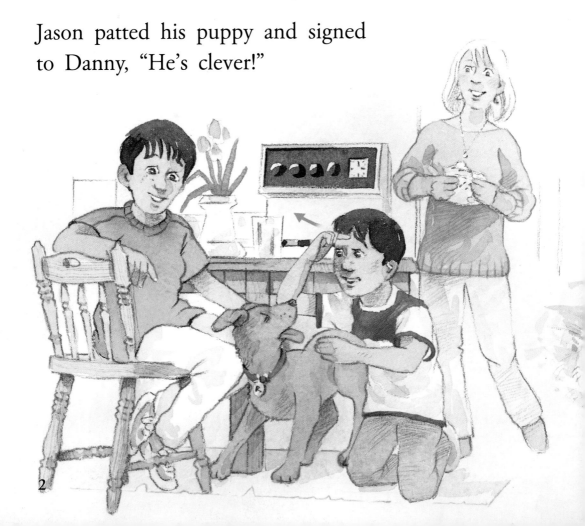

Mom smiled and said, "I'm pleased about that! He's getting so big, and I don't want him crashing into things and breaking them! Take him out to his cage now, Jason. Aunt Kathy and little Devon will be here soon, and Devon might be afraid of dogs."

With Rocky safely in his cage, Jason opened the gate for Aunt Kathy and Devon and waited for them to come up the long driveway.

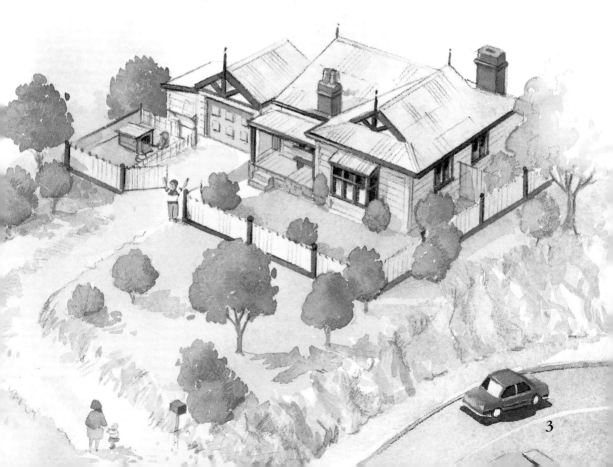

Danny and Jason took Devon to see Rocky.

"Look, Rocky! Here's Rabbit!" said Devon, as he showed his toy to the dog.

"Rocky is blind!" Jason said.

"Jason's puppy can't see," Danny explained.

Rocky stood in front of Devon and sniffed him and the toy.

"Puppy likes me," Devon laughed, "and Rabbit, too!"

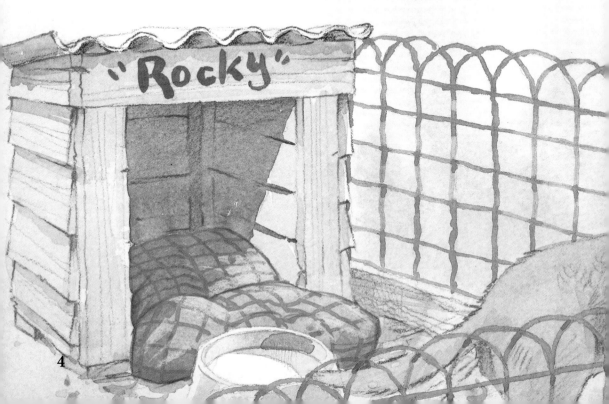

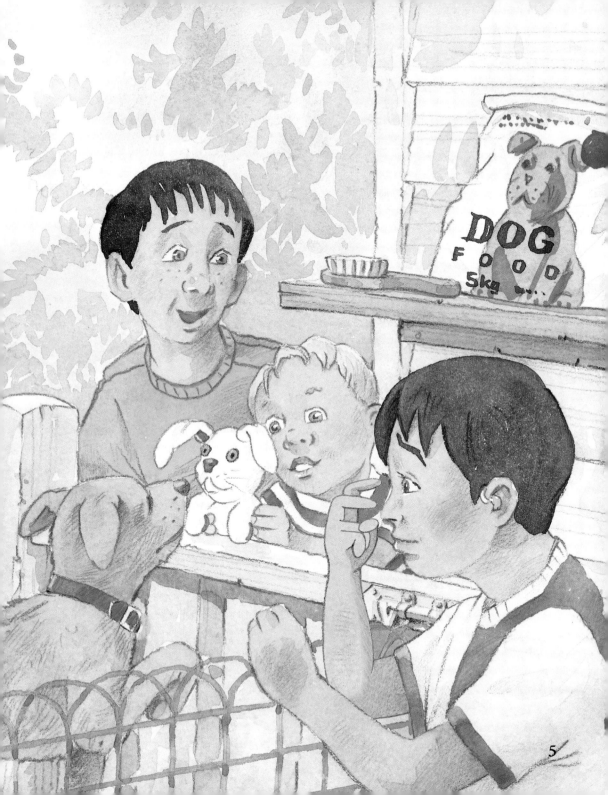

Where Is Devon?

When lunch was over, Devon went to sleep on Jason's bed while Mom and Aunt Kathy and the boys played a card game.

After the card game, Aunt Kathy challenged the boys to a board game. "I'll take a peek at Devon before we start," she said.

Aunt Kathy came out of the bedroom and cried, "He's not there!"

"Oh," said Mom, "he must have gone outside!"

"He might be talking to Rocky!" signed Jason.

"I hope so!" Mom replied.

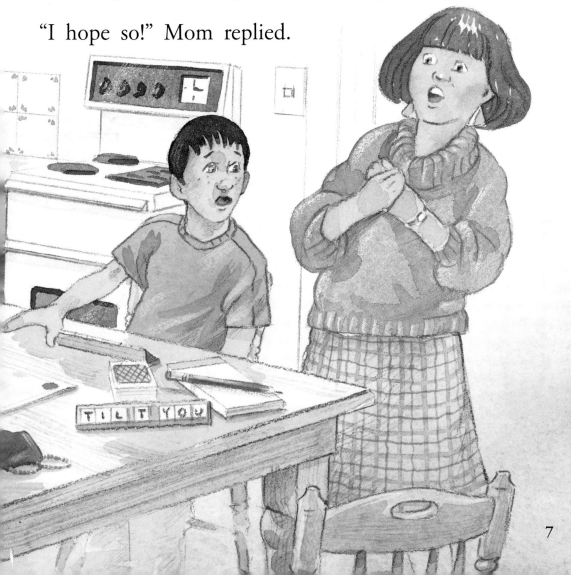

Outside, Devon was nowhere to be seen.

"The gate!" Jason signed. "I forgot to shut the gate!"

"We all forgot to shut the gate," Mom said gently. "I'm sure he'll be here somewhere."

Aunt Kathy looked frightened.

"Don't worry, Aunt Kathy," Jason said slowly, "we'll find him."

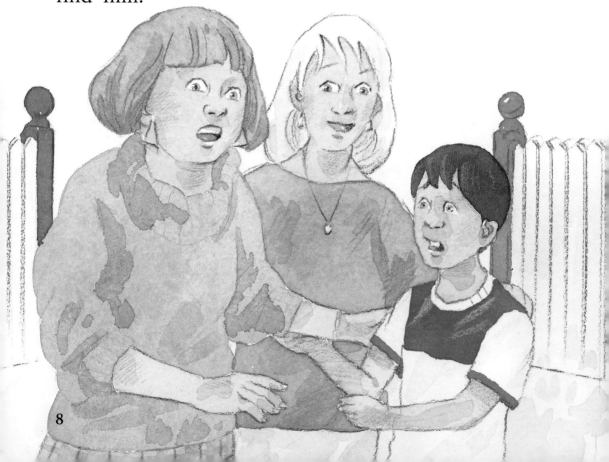

Chapter 3
Searching!

Danny and Jason searched the yard while Mom and Aunt Kathy looked inside the house.

"He couldn't have gone far," said Mom. "He's never wandered away before, and I'm sure we would have noticed him going outside. You keep looking here, Kathy, and the boys and I will search the driveway. If we can't find him, we'll call the police."

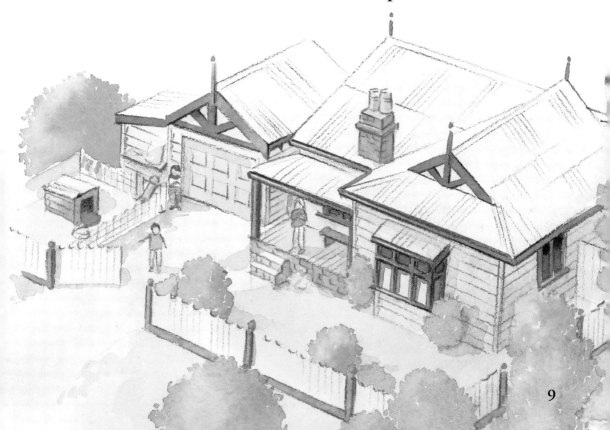

Jason put Rocky on a leash and waited at the gate. Mom and Danny joined him, and they walked down the driveway. "Devon! Devon!" they called.

While Mom kept calling, Jason and Danny searched under the trees along the driveway. Soon they were at the road.

"Oh, Mom!" cried Danny. "What if he came out here? He's too little to be near this dangerous road."

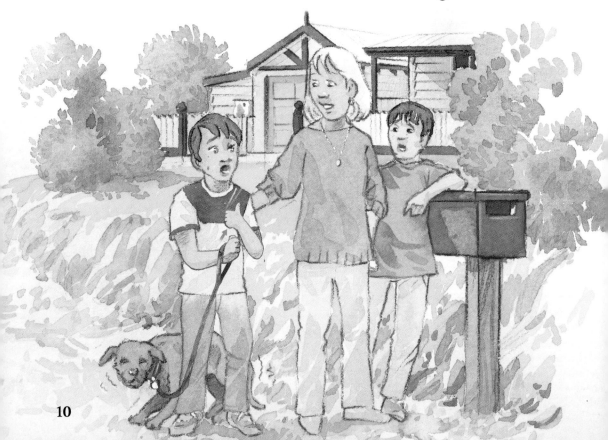

"Rocky is too little to be out here, too," signed Jason. "Look at him! He's afraid because he can't see what is making all the noise."

"Take him home, Jason," Mom said. "Danny and I'll look up the road. You and Rocky go back to Aunt Kathy and take another look inside the house."

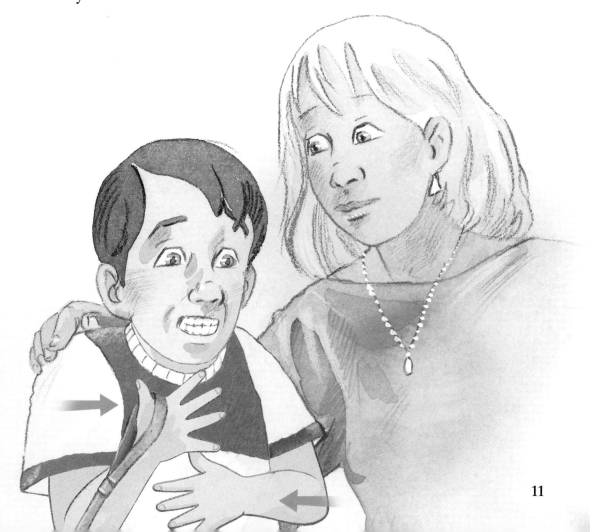

Chapter
4
Great Detectives!

Jason and Rocky found Aunt Kathy sitting on the steps. She looked up at Jason and cried, "He can't just disappear! What's happened to him?"

Jason said, "Rocky and I'll take another look inside, Aunt Kathy."

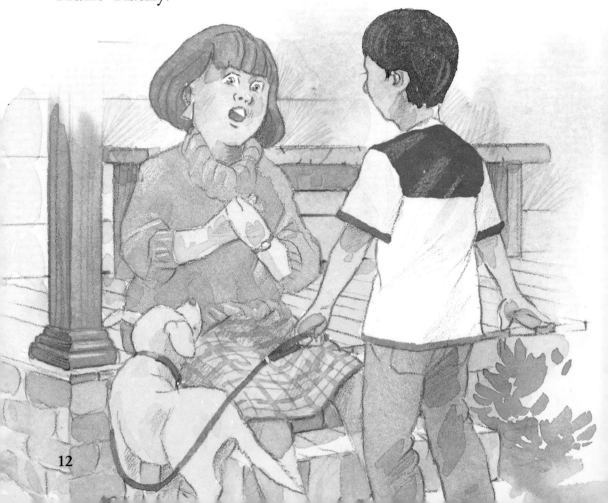

When he and Rocky got to his bedroom, Jason saw Devon's toy rabbit on the floor.

"Oh!" he thought. "Devon never goes anywhere without his rabbit. He must be here somewhere!"

Rocky barked, sniffed the rabbit, and then put his head under Jason's bed. Jason crouched down to look under the bed, too, and there was Devon, fast asleep, his yellow blanket in his hands.

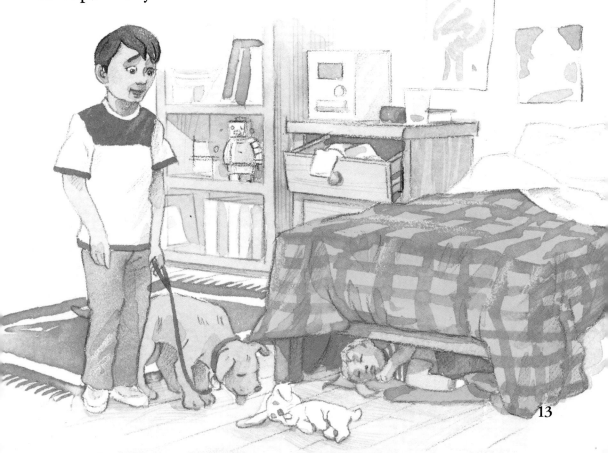

Jason and Rocky rushed outside. Mom and Danny were back, and Mom had her arms around Aunt Kathy. Jason signed quickly to Mom and Danny.

"He's here, Kathy!" Mom shouted. "He's under the bed!"

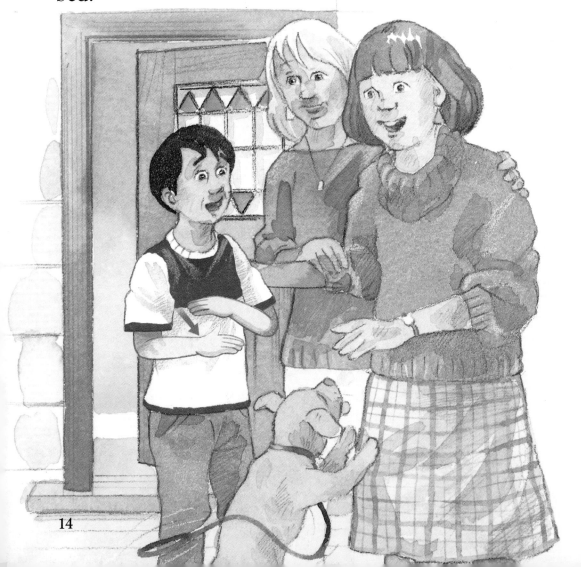

Mom, Danny, and Aunt Kathy followed Jason to his bedroom.

Aunt Kathy moved the bed and lifted Devon up. She hugged him tightly and turned to Jason.

"Oh, thank you, Jason!" she said. "You were so clever to find him!"

"Rocky and I both found him," Jason laughed.

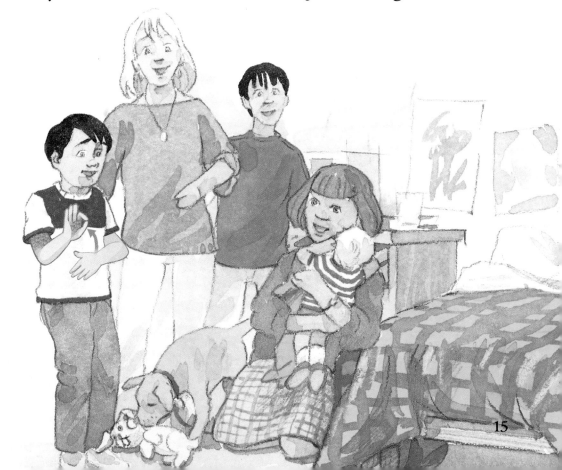

Then Jason turned to Mom and Danny and signed excitedly. "I saw the rabbit, and Rocky could smell Devon. We didn't need the police today! Rocky and I are great detectives because I use my eyes to find the clues, and Rocky uses his nose."

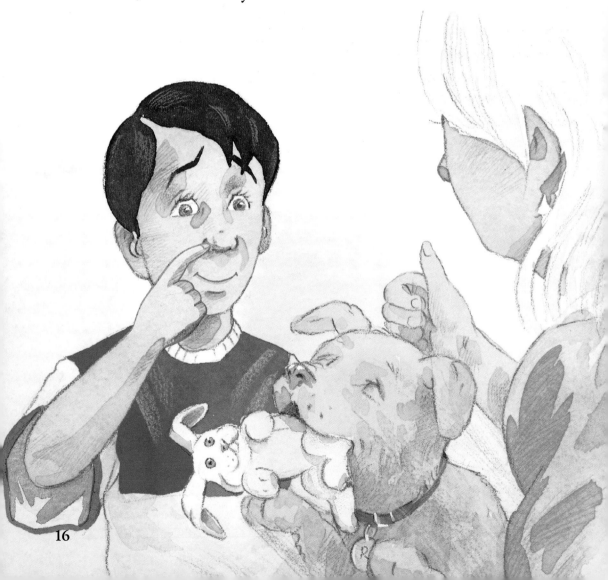